D0894302

Econ.

SCOPE AND STANDARDS OF ADDICTIONS NURSING PRACTICE

WITHDRAWN

nurses
books
.org
The Publishing Program of ANA

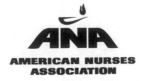

ANA
AMERICAN NURSES ASSOCIATION

Washington, D.C.
2004

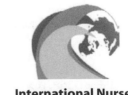

International Nurses Society on Addictions

Library of Congress Cataloging-in-Publication data

International Nurses Society on Addictions.
  Scope and standards of addictions nursing practice / International
Nurses Society on Addictions, American Nurses Association.—
  p. ; cm.
Rev. ed. of: Standards of addictions nursing practice with selected
diagnoses and criteria / American Nurses' Association and National
Nurses Society on Addictions. c1988.
Includes bibliographical references.
  ISBN 1-55810-218-3
1. Substance abuse—Nursing—Standards. 2. Psychiatric
nursing—Standards.
[DNLM: 1. Nursing Care—standards. 2. Substance-Related
Disorders—nursing. 3. Evidence-Based Medicine. 4. Nursing Assessment.
5. Nursing Diagnosis. WY 160 I595s 2004] I. American Nurses
Association. II. National Nurses Society on Addictions (U.S.) Standards
of addictions nursing practice with selected diagnoses and criteria.
III. Title.

RC564.A516 2004
616.89'0231—dc22

                              2004001780

The American Nurses Association (ANA) is a national professional association. This ANA publication—*Scope and Standards of Addictions Nursing Practice, Second Edition*—reflects the thinking of the nursing profession on various issues and should be reviewed in conjunction with state board of nursing policies and practices. State law, rules, and regulations govern the practice of nursing, while *Scope and Standards of Addictions Nursing Practice, Second Edition* guides nurses in the application of their professional skills and responsibilities.

Published by nursesbooks.org
The Publishing Program of ANA

American Nurses Association
600 Maryland Avenue, SW • Suite 100 West • Washington, DC 20024
1-800-274-4ANA • http://www.nursingworld.org/

ISBN 1-55810-218-3
04SSAN   2M   03/04

ᴸ
ᵢ16
04

Acknowledgements

The International Nurses Society on Addictions (IntNSA) is grateful to the following individuals who have put their time, energy, and commitment into the completion of this revised 2003 version of the *Scope and Standards of Addictions Nursing*. IntNSA wishes to thank the ANA for its contributions to the completion of this important document and the support of the IntNSA Board of Directors.

Editors/Chairs of Revision
Karen Allen, PhD, RN, FAAN, Andrews University
Diane Snow, PhD, APRN, BC, CARN, PMHNP, University of Texas at Arlington
*Lynette Jack, PhD, RN, CARN, University of Pittsburgh

Other contributors and reviewers
Merry Armstrong, DNSc, MS, ARNP
 Carolyn Baird, MEd, RNC-PMH, CARN-AP, CAAP
*Kathleen Ballard, MSN, RN
*Cass Breslin, RN
 Janice Feigenbaum, PhD, RN
*Kathleen Flanagan, RN
*Kem Louie, PhD, RN, APRN, BC, FAAN
*Connie Mele, MSN, RN, CARN-AP
 Dana Murphy Parker, MS, RN
 Christine Savage, Ph.D, RN
*Eleanor Sullivan, PhD, RN, FAAN
 *Lynn Swisher, PhD, RN
*Nancy Fisk, MSN, RN
*Patricia Rowell, PhD, RN

Members of original revision workgroup.

CONTENTS

Acknowledgements   iii

Practice Standards for Addictions Nursing   vi

Scope of Practice for Addictions Nursing   1

Introduction   1

Extent of the Addictions Problem   2

    Incidence and Prevalence of Alcohol and Other Drug Addictions   2

    Incidence and Prevalence of Alcohol and Other Drug Addictions   4
     Worldwide

    Incidence and Prevalence of Other Addictions   5

    Addicted Patients in Clinical Settings   5

Description of Addictions   5

    Definition and Characteristics   5

    Process of Addiction   7

    Diagnosing Addiction   9

The Continuum of Care for Addictions Nursing   10

    Prevention   10

    Early Intervention (Brief Interventions)   11

    Treatment   12

    Recovery and Relapse Prevention   14

Description of Addictions Nursing   14

    Phenomena of Concern   16

    Special Diagnostic Phenomena   21

    Specialty Practice: Generalist Level   21

    Specialty Practice: Advanced Level   23

    Additional Activities of Addictions Nurses   24

    Education for Addictions Nursing Practice   26

    Certification   27

    Implications for Research   28

    Peer Assistance   29

Standards of Care for Addictions Nursing   31

Standard 1. Assessment   31

Standard 2. Diagnosis   33

Standard 3. Outcome Identification   35

Standard 4. Planning   36

Standard 5. Implementation   37

    Standard 5a. Therapeutic Alliance   37

    Standard 5b. Health Teaching   38

    Standard 5c. Self-Care and Self-Management   39

    Standard 5d. Pharmacological, Biological, and Complementary Therapies   40

    Standard 5e. Therapeutic Milieu   41

    Standard 5f. Counseling   42

Standard 6. Evaluation   43

Standards of Professional Performance for Addictions Nursing   **45**
Standard 7. Quality of Care   45
Standard 8. Performance Appraisal   46
Standard 9. Education   47
Standard 10. Collegiality   48
Standard 11. Ethics   49
Standard 12. Collaboration   50
Standard 13. Research   51
Standard 14. Resource Utilization   52

Advanced Practice Standards of Care for Addictions Nursing   **53**
Standard 1. Assessment   53
Standard 2. Diagnosis   53
Standard 3. Outcome Identification   54
Standard 4. Planning   54
Standard 5. Implementation   55
    Standard 5a. Case Management and Coordination of Care   55
    Standard 5b. Consultation   56
    Standard 5c. Health Promotion, Health Maintenance,   56
      and Health Teaching
    Standard 5d. Prescriptive Authority and Treatment   57
    Standard 5e. Psychotherapy and Complementary Therapy   58
    Standard 5f. Referral   58
Standard 6. Evaluation   59

Advanced Practice Standards of Professional Performance   **61**
  for Addictions Nursing
Standard 7. Quality of Care   61
Standard 8. Self-Evaluation   62
Standard 9. Education   62
Standard 10. Leadership   63
Standard 11. Ethics   63
Standard 12. Interdisciplinary Process   64
Standard 13. Research   64

Glossary   **65**

References   **69**

Appendix A. Specific Prevention Strategies   **77**

Appendix B. Motivational Interventions   **79**

Appendix C. Code of Ethics for Addictions Nurses   **81**

Index   **83**

PRACTICE STANDARDS FOR ADDICTIONS NURSING: STANDARDS OF CARE

STANDARD 1. ASSESSMENT

The addictions nurse collects patient health data.

STANDARD 2. DIAGNOSIS

The addictions nurse analyzes the assessment data in determining diagnoses.

STANDARD 3. OUTCOME IDENTIFICATION

The addictions nurse identifies expected outcomes individualized to the patient.

STANDARD 4. PLANNING

The addictions nurse develops an individualized plan of care that prescribes interventions to attain expected outcomes.

STANDARD 5. IMPLEMENTATION

The addictions nurse implements the interventions identified in the plan of care.

STANDARD 5A. THERAPEUTIC ALLIANCE

The addictions nurse uses the "therapeutic self" to establish a therapeutic alliance with the patient and to structure nursing interventions to promote development of insight, coping skills, and motivation for change in behavior that promotes health.

STANDARD 5B. HEALTH TEACHING

The addictions nurse, through health teaching, assists individuals, families, groups, and communities in achieving satisfying, productive, and healthy patterns of living.

STANDARD 5C. SELF-CARE AND SELF-MANAGEMENT

The addictions nurse uses the knowledge and philosophy of self-care and self-management to assist the patient in learning new ways to address stress, maintain self-control, accept personal responsibility, and integrate healthy coping behaviors into life-style choices.

STANDARD 5D. PHARMACOLOGICAL, BIOLOGICAL, AND COMPLEMENTARY THERAPIES

The addictions nurse applies knowledge of pharmacological, biological, and complementary therapies and uses clinical skills to restore the patient's health and prevent consequences from addiction.

STANDARD 5E. THERAPEUTIC MILIEU

The addictions nurse structures, provides, and maintains a therapeutic environment in collaboration with the patient and other healthcare providers.

STANDARD 5F. COUNSELING

The addictions nurse uses counseling interventions to assist patients in promoting healthy coping abilities, preventing addiction, and addressing issues related to patterns of abuse and addiction.

STANDARD 6. EVALUATION

The addictions nurse evaluates the patient's progress toward attainment of expected outcomes.

PRACTICE STANDARDS
FOR ADDICTIONS NURSING:
STANDARDS OF PROFESSIONAL PERFORMANCE

STANDARD 7. QUALITY OF CARE

The addictions nurse systematically evaluates the quality of care and effectiveness of nursing practice.

STANDARD 8. PERFORMANCE APPRAISAL

The addictions nurse evaluates his or her own nursing practice in relation to professional practice standards and relevant statutes and regulations.

STANDARD 9. EDUCATION

The addictions nurse acquires and maintains current knowledge and competency in nursing practice.

STANDARD 10. COLLEGIALITY

The addictions nurse interacts with and contributes to the professional development of peers, and treats other healthcare providers as colleagues.

STANDARD 11. ETHICS

The addictions nurse's decisions and actions on behalf of patients are determined and implemented in an ethical manner.

STANDARD 12. COLLABORATION

The addictions nurse collaborates with the patient, significant others, and other healthcare providers in providing patient care.

STANDARD 13. RESEARCH

The addictions nurse uses theory and evidence from research findings to guide practice.

STANDARD 14. RESOURCE UTILIZATION

The addictions nurse considers factors related to safety, effectiveness, and cost in planning and delivering patient care.

Advanced Practice Standards for Addictions Nursing: Standards of Care

STANDARD 1. ASSESSMENT

The advanced practice addictions registered nurse collects comprehensive patient health data.

STANDARD 2. DIAGNOSIS

The advanced practice addictions registered nurse critically analyzes the assessment data in determining the diagnoses.

STANDARD 3. OUTCOME IDENTIFICATION

The advanced practice registered nurse identifies expected outcomes derived from the assessment data and diagnoses, and individualizes expected outcomes with the patient and the healthcare team when appropriate.

STANDARD 4. PLANNING

The advanced practice addictions registered nurse develops a comprehensive treatment plan that includes interventions to attain expected outcomes.

STANDARD 5. IMPLEMENTATION

The advanced practice addictions registered nurse prescribes, orders, or implements addictions interventions and treatments for the plan of care.

STANDARD 5A. CASE MANAGEMENT AND COORDINATION OF CARE

The advanced practice addictions registered nurse provides comprehensive clinical coordination of care and case management.

STANDARD 5B. CONSULTATION

The advanced practice addictions registered nurse provides consultation to influence the plan of care for patients, enhance the abilities of others to provide quality care to addicted patients, and effect change in the system.

STANDARD 5C. HEALTH PROMOTION, HEALTH MAINTENANCE, AND HEALTH TEACHING

The advanced practice addictions registered nurse employs complex strategies, interventions, and teaching to promote, maintain, and improve health and prevent illness and injury.

STANDARD 5D. PRESCRIPTIVE AUTHORITY AND TREATMENT

The advanced practice addictions registered nurse uses prescriptive authority, procedures, and treatments in accordance with educational preparation, state and federal laws and regulations, applicable nurse practice acts, and appropriate advanced practice certification to treat illness and improve functional health status or to provide preventive care.

STANDARD 5E. PSYCHOTHERAPY AND COMPLEMENTARY THERAPY

The advanced practice addictions registered nurse conducts individual, group, and family psychotherapy, and educates about and evaluates the use of complementary therapies to promote healthy lifestyles, prevent addictive behaviors, treat addictions and improve health status and functional abilities.

STANDARD 5F. REFERRAL

The advanced practice addictions registered nurse identifies the need for additional care and makes referrals as needed.

STANDARD 6. EVALUATION

The advanced practice addictions registered nurse evaluates the patient's progress in attaining expected outcomes.

ADVANCED PRACTICE STANDARDS FOR ADDICTIONS NURSING: STANDARDS OF PROFESSIONAL PERFORMANCE

STANDARD 7. QUALITY OF CARE

The advanced practice addictions registered nurse develops criteria for and evaluates the quality of care and effectiveness of advanced practice addictions registered nurses.

STANDARD 8. SELF-EVALUATION

The advanced practice addictions registered nurse continuously evaluates their nursing practice in relation to professional practice standards and relevant statutes and regulations, and is accountable to the public and to the profession for providing competent clinical care.

STANDARD 9. EDUCATION

The advanced practice addictions registered nurse acquires and maintains current knowledge and skills in addictions practice.

STANDARD 10. LEADERSHIP

The advanced practice addictions registered nurse serves as a leader and a role model for the professional development of peers, colleagues, and others.

STANDARD 11. ETHICS

The advanced practice addictions registered nurse integrates ethical principles and norms in all areas of practice.

STANDARD 12. INTERDISCIPLINARY PROCESS

The advanced practice addictions registered nurse promotes an interdisciplinary process in providing patient care.

STANDARD 13. RESEARCH

The advanced practice addictions registered nurse utilizes theory and research to discover, examine, and evaluate knowledge, theories, and creative approaches to healthcare practice.

SCOPE OF PRACTICE
FOR ADDICTIONS NURSING

Introduction

In 1983 the American Nurses Association, the National Nurses Society on Addictions, and the Drug and Alcohol Nurses Association led the effort to delineate the practice of addictions nursing by forming a task force on addictions nursing practice. This resulted in the publication of *Care of Clients with Addictions: Dimensions of Nursing Practice*, which described nursing practice in the prevention and intervention of abuse and addiction of substances and behaviors (American Nurses Association, Drug and Alcohol Nursing Association, & National Nurses Society on Addictions, 1987). In 1989 the *Standards of Addiction Nursing Practice with Selected Diagnoses and Criteria* was published by the National Nurses Society on Addiction and the American Nurses Association. Addictions nursing practice is a distinct specialty that integrates biological, behavioral, environmental, psychological, social, cultural, and spiritual aspects of human responses to the illness of addiction into the nursing care provided to those affected by this disorder/disease, regardless of the clinical setting.

Since that time, significant changes occurring within the healthcare arena have affected addictions nursing practice including:

- Research on the causes and treatment of addictions revealing new insights that affect the care of addicted persons.

- Social and healthcare policy that affects the prevention and treatment of addiction in individuals and populations.

- Healthcare financing and reimbursement that help shape when, where, how, and what kind of care addicted persons receive.

- Graying of the population, which has meant adapting and developing modalities of care that meet the specific needs of older individuals (this includes the need for tools for assessing substance use and abuse).

Like other nursing specialties, the scope of addictions nursing practice continues to evolve. Society's increasing need and demand for nurses with expertise in the treatment and prevention of addictions has broadened the scope of the specialty. As nursing moves toward an evidence-based model of practice, the specialty of addictions nursing is growing in its knowledge about addictions and its development of addictions theories and theories from related disciplines.

With the increasing prevalence of substance use disorders and other addictions in all segments of the population, all nurses, regardless of their practice setting, require evidence-based standards of care for their patients affected directly or indirectly by addictions. The specialty of addictions nursing provides leadership to the profession by providing evidence-based standards of care, cutting edge nursing research related to addiction, and forums for developing new and innovative approaches aimed at reducing the prevalence of addiction and increasing the use of effective interventions related to addiction.

Extent of the Addictions Problem

Incidence and Prevalence of Alcohol and Other Drug Addictions

Based on the most recent data from the National Household Survey on Drug Abuse (SAMHSA, 2002, pp. 1–4) in the United States:

- 109 million Americans age 12 years and older reported current use of alcohol, meaning they used alcohol at least once during the 30 days prior to the interview.

- 25.1 million Americans aged 12 years and older reported driving under the influence of alcohol at least once in the 12 months prior to the interview. Approximately 22.8% of young adults age 18 to 25 years drove under the influence of alcohol.

- 10.1 million current drinkers were age 12–20, despite the fact that alcohol consumption is not legal for those Americans under 21 years of age. Of this group, 6.8 million engaged in binge drinking with 2.1 million classified as heavy drinkers.

- An estimated 66.5 million Americans age 12 years and older reported use of a tobacco product during the 30 days prior to the interview.

- Approximately 13.0% of youth age 12 to 17 years used a tobacco product during the 30 days prior to the interview. However, based on the *Monitoring the Future* study, Johnston et al. (2003, p. 42) reported that 31.4% of eighth graders, 47.4% of tenth graders, and 57.2% of twelfth graders had smoked cigarettes at least once in their life.

- An estimated 15.9 million Americans age 12 years and older (7.1 % of this population) used an illicit drug at least once during the 30 days prior to the interview. Approximately 10.8 % of 12- to 17-year-olds and 18.8 % of young adults ages 18 to 25 years used an illicit drug at least once during the 30 days prior to the interview.

- Approximately 1.6% of Americans age 12 years and older have engaged in the nonmedical use of pain relievers and 0.6 % have engaged in the nonmedical use of tranquilizers.

- Approximately 8.1 million Americans age 12 and older have tried ecstasy (MDMA) at least once in their life.

- Close to one million (957,000) Americans age 12 years and older reported the use of Oxycontin for a nonmedical purpose.

- An estimated 16.6 million persons age 12 years and older were classified with dependence on or abuse of either alcohol or illicit drugs (7.3 % of the population).

- Based on the *Monitoring the Future* study, Johnston et al. (2003) reported that 24.5% of eighth graders, 44.6% of tenth graders, and 53.0% of twelfth graders in the United States had used an illicit drug at least once in their life. This use included:

  - 19.2% of eighth graders, 38.7% of tenth graders, and 47.8% of twelfth graders had used marijuana or hashish.

  - 15.2% of eighth graders, 13.5% of tenth graders, and 11.7% of twelfth graders had used an inhalant.

  - 4.1% of eighth graders, 7.8% of tenth graders, and 12.0% of twelfth graders had used a hallucinogen.

  - 3.1% of twelfth graders used PCP (phencyclidine).

  - 4.3% of eighth graders, 6.6% of tenth graders, and 10.5% of twelfth graders had used ecstasy (MDMA).

  - 3.6% of eighth graders, 6.1% of tenth graders, and 7.8% of twelfth graders had used cocaine or crack.

  - 1.6% of eighth graders, 1.8% of tenth graders, and 1.7% of twelfth graders had used heroin.

  - 10.1% of twelfth graders had used a narcotic other than heroi.

  - 8.7% of eighth graders, 14.9% of tenth graders, and 16.8% of twelfth graders had used an amphetamine.

  - 3.5% of eighth graders, 6.1% of tenth graders, and 6.7% of twelfth graders had used a methamphetamine.

  - 9.5% of twelfth graders had used a barbiturate.

  - 4.3% of eighth graders, 8.8% of tenth graders, and 11.4% of twelfth graders had used a tranquilizer.

  - 0.8% of eighth graders, and 1.3% of tenth graders had used rohypnol.

- The problems of abuse and dependence among the older population are believed to be substantial, but difficult to estimate because of the lack of data and focus on this issue (Korper & Council, 2002).

- Korper and Raskin (Korper & Council, 2002) project a doubling of individuals age 50 years and older with substance abuse problems in the next 20 years.

- An estimated 14.8 million American adults age 18 years or older had a severe mental illness (7.3% of the population). An estimated 3.0 million people, approximately 20.3% of this group, were dependent on or abused alcohol or illicit drugs (SAMHSA, 2002, p. 4).

Incidence and Prevalence of Alcohol and Other Drug Addictions Worldwide

The Global Burden of Disease (GBD), a project of the World Health Organization (WHO) and the World Bank (Murray & Lopez, 1996), highlighted the significance of the burden of mental health and addiction issues by estimating disability rather than more traditional mortality rates. Based on estimates of the Disease Adjusted Life Years (DALYs) in 1990, psychiatric conditions, including substance misuse, accounted for nearly 11% of disease burden worldwide. In the developed regions of the world alcohol use was the leading cause of disability in males and the tenth largest in women. In developing regions alcohol use was the fourth largest cause of disability in men.

Projections for the year 2020 in the GBD include a dramatic rise in deaths from tobacco, which is expected to kill more people than any single disease, and which will surpass the HIV epidemic. From its 1990 level of 2.6% of all disease burdens worldwide, the burden from diseases related to tobacco is expected to be up to 9%. Tobacco is fast becoming a global health emergency.

Violence will rise from 19th place to 12th place, and HIV is expected to be the 10th leading cause of disease burden worldwide by 2020. Closely associated with drug and alcohol use is the number of road traffic accidents, which will rise from 9th to 3rd place in young adults. Unipolar major depression, often a sequela or etiological factor for abuse and addiction, is expected to be the leading cause of disease burden in women and in developing countries, while overall it is projected to be ranked second worldwide, accounting for 5.7% of the disease burden in 2020.

Incidence and Prevalence of Other Addictions

According to the National Gambling Impact and Policy Commission (NGIPC) (1999), gambling is an increasingly popular leisure activity enjoyed in the United States by a majority of adults and youth. There is an estimated 1 to 3% prevalence rate of adult problem or pathological gambling, with a 3:1 gender ratio of men to women (APA, 2000). Blume (1997) reported that approximately 4% of adults have some gambling related problems, with a higher rate of 9% for compulsive gambling among those in treatment for addictive substance disorders. Some experts place the problem gambling rate among adolescents to be higher (Adlaf & Ialomiteanu, 2000; Jacobs, 2000) The NGIPC (1999) study estimated that the prevalence rate of pathological gambling of adolescents is approximately 5%, while the rate of problem gambling is approximately 6%.

The prevalence of sexual addiction has been estimated at 3 to 6% of the American population (Goodman, 1997). Many regard eating disorders as food addiction, or the use of food in an addictive behavioral manner to address emotional issues (Blundell & Hill, 1993; David & Claridge, 1998; Pirke, 1990). Approximately 0.5% of women between the ages of 15 and 40 years exhibit anorexia. One to 1.5% of women exhibit symptoms of bulimia (Gold, Johnson, and Stennie, 1997).

Addicted Patients in Clinical Settings

Based on data from the 1998 National Hospital Discharge Survey, Hall and Popovich (2000) reported that approximately 1.5% of discharges from short-stay hospitals gave alcohol-related diagnoses as the first-listed diagnosis. This value would be much higher if tallied from any listed diagnoses. Evaluating alcohol-related discharge diagnoses does not account for conditions such as peptic ulcer disease, burns, fractures, and injuries from automobile accidents that commonly have alcohol as a contributory factor (National Institute on Alcohol Abuse and Alcoholism, 1998). Nurses in other healthcare facilities care for the untold numbers of patients with addictions-related illness resulting from drug abuse/addiction, eating disorders, and lifestyle illnesses, such as HIV/AIDS obtained through addictive behaviors.

Description of Addictions

Definition and Characteristics

In the past ten years researchers, under the auspices of the National Institute on Drug Abuse and the National Institute on Alcohol Abuse and Alcoholism, have repeatedly demonstrated that addiction is a brain disorder/disease. Specific neurochemical processes occurring in the brain are linked to addiction and relapse in individuals attempting to maintain abstinence. The scientific evidence has helped to remove the former belief that individuals with an addiction suffered from a moral deficit or insufficient willpower. What is now known is that the development of an addictive disorder is related to a complex interaction of environmental, social, genetic, psychological, and biological risk factors (Wilcox & Erickson, 2000).

Current research is helping us to understand the mechanism by which exposure to chemicals results in addiction. According to the National Institute on Drug Abuse (1994), prolonged exposure to drugs leads to molecular adaptations in certain proteins found within neurons in the mesocorticolimbic dopamine system—a brain pathway that is important for drug reward and craving. Dopamine, produced from the precursor tyrosine, is dysregulated as the disease progresses. The medial forebrain bundle, comprising the ventral tegmental area, lateral hypothalamus, nucleus accumbens, amygdala, and frontal cortex, is involved in addiction/dependency from the excessive dopamine release. Thus, the person with an addiction has a drive that is "automatic" and outside of conscious control (Wilcox & Erickson, 2000). Other neurotranmsitters involved include serotonin (5HT) and gamma amino butyric acid (GABA). Long-term adaptations in these proteins caused by chronic drug use may contribute to such addictive aspects as: tolerance, sensitization, reinforcement, and the compulsion to continue to achieve a desired effect.

Addiction is an illness characterized by compulsion, loss of control, and continued use despite perceived negative consequences. Types of addictions include alcohol dependence (alcoholism), drug dependence (including nicotine), eating disorders, excessive gambling or spending, and compulsive sexual disorders. Addiction is progressive, but does respond to comprehensive and varied treatment approaches, which foster the patient's active participation and acceptance of responsibility.

Addiction is a complex neurobiobehavioral disorder characterized by impaired control, compulsive use, dependency, and craving for the activity, substance, or food. Relapses are possible even after long periods of abstinence (National Institute on Drug Abuse [NIDA], 2002b; Wilcox & Erickson, 2000). Addiction is often (but not always) accompanied by physiological dependence, consisting of a withdrawal syndrome, or tolerance (NIDA, 2002a). Factors contributing to the development of addiction include genetic predisposition, the reinforcing properties and access to the substance, food, or activity, family and peer influences, sociocultural environment, personality, and existing psychiatric disorders (Goldstein, 1994). The terms *addictive disorder* and *addiction* are used interchangeably (Armstrong, Feigenbaum, Savage, Snow & Vourakis, 2005). Addiction is an illness that causes major impairment, but which will respond to comprehensive and varied treatment approaches which foster the patient's active participation and acceptance of responsibility.

Addiction is multidimensional, with multiple causes. One model that explains the etiology of addiction is the *biopsychosocial model* (Allen, 1996). In this explanation, addiction develops as a result of one or a combination of the following:

- Biological vulnerability (including neurochemical, genetic, and hereditary)
- Environmental vulnerability and exposure to risk factors (in utero exposure, etc.)
- Access to substances or activities (e.g. gambling)
- Predisposition to addictive behaviors and reinforcement when using/abusing
- Enabling behaviors by the individuals and systems around the person
- Environmental, cultural, or community influences, and learning processes

Addiction represents only one end of a continuum where problems associated with the use of addictive substances or behaviors are the most severe and disabling. However, there are other points on the continuum, including low risk, at risk, problem use/misuse/abuse, and dependence where intervention can occur based on the stage of change and level of motivation to change (CSAT: SAMHSA, 1997).

Process of Addiction

The U.S. Substance Abuse and Mental Health Services Administration's (SAMHSA) Center for Substance Abuse Treatment (SAMHSA, 1994) describes the five stages of the process of addiction:

1. Experimental/social use
2. Problem use/misuse/abuse
3. Dependency/addiction
4. Recovery
5. Relapse

For some persons it is progressive in nature and may not be linear in sequence. Other persons may not progress to a level of dependence, and current research focuses on the genetic predisposition to the disease as necessary to progress to dependence. Persons with a family history of alcohol or other drug dependency are at high risk for developing addiction or dependence. However, all persons should be screened periodically and routinely for substance use disorders (Snow, 2000a) and other types of addiction, e.g., eating disorders and gambling.

In the *experimentation/low risk/at risk* stage of the addiction process, engaging in the addictive behavior occurs occasionally, with friends or family, to satisfy curiosity, give in to peer pressure, obtain social acceptance, relieve boredom, produce feelings of pleasure, or diminish social inhibitions. The person experiences it as fun, exciting, and being in control. There is little or no change evident in any aspect of life.

In the *problem use/misuse/abuse* stage of the addiction process, engaging in the addictive behavior occurs on a more regular basis—which may be several times per week. The behaviors begin to occur when the person is alone, and include preoccupation and planning for resources, places, and times when the behavior will occur. The behavior is engaged in to manipulate emotions, cope with stress, and relieve uncomfortable feelings, such as depression or withdrawal, when not involved with the addictive behavior. The effects at this stage include euphoria, stress reduction, guilt, shame, fear, unsuccessful tries at controlling the situation, and the need for more of the behavior to produce the desired effects. Behavioral indications of a problem include a decline in school or work performance, mood swings, personality changes, change in friendships, etc.

In the *dependency/addiction* stage, use of the addictive behavior is continual and out of control. The person will use any means necessary to obtain what is needed to participate in the addictive behavior, including engaging in criminal activity and taking serious risks, to avoid pain and depression as well as to escape from the realities of life. Unfortunately the effect provided at this stage is a constant state of pain (physical or emotional) or discomfort, depression, aggression, irritation, apathy, focused on seeking normalcy. Some individuals may experience suicidal thoughts or attempts and some may experience blackouts. Physical deterioration is evidenced in weight loss and health problems, poor appearance, volatile mood swings. The individual is frequently absent from home or work, lacks concern about being caught, and is just concerned about being able to engage in addictive behavior.

During *recovery*, the person experiences a remission, where the addictive behavior is discontinued. Dramatic lifestyle changes occur and their effects are evident in personal and professional aspects of life. However, the chance for a relapse with the return to the previous addiction state and the person's life again being out of control remains. (SAMHSA, 1994)

During the *relapse* phase, there has been a re-occurrence of symptoms of dependence/addiction.

Diagnosing Addiction

Nurses practicing in any clinical setting will encounter patients exhibiting symptoms that point to addiction. As providers of holistic, effective, and safe care, nurses need to be aware of their role in clarifying their suspicions with an assessment and then referring patients for appropriate diagnosis and care.

One of the significant changes in the addictions field is the increased clarity in symptoms used for diagnosing problem use/substance abuse and addiction/substance dependence. *Diagnostic and Statistical Manual of Mental Disorders, 4th Edition Text Revision* (DSM-IV-TR; American Psychiatric Association, 2000) presents the criteria for diagnosing problem use/substance abuse: a maladaptive pattern of the behavior exists to the point that clinically significant impairment or distress, as manifested by one or more of the following, occurs within a 12-month period:

- Recurrent participation in the behavior results in a failure to fulfill major role obligations at work, school, or home.

- Recurrent participation in the behavior occurs in situations in which it is physically hazardous.

- Recurrent participation in the behavior leads to legal problems

- Participation in the behavior continues despite persistent social or interpersonal problems caused or exacerbated by the effects of the addictive behavior.

The diagnosis of substance dependency/addiction occurs when three or more or more of the following occur within a 12-month period:

- Tolerance: either a markedly increased intake of the substance is needed to achieve the same effect *or* with continued use, the same amount of the substance has markedly less effect.

- Withdrawal: the substance's characteristic withdrawal syndrome is experienced or the substance (or one closely related) is used to avoid or relieve withdrawal symptoms.

- The amount or duration of use is often greater than intended.
- The patient repeatedly tries without success to control or reduce substance use.
- The patient spends much time using the substance, recovering from its effects, or trying to obtain it.
- The patient reduces or abandons important work, social, or leisure activities because of substance abuse.
- The patient continues to use the substance, despite knowing that it has probably caused ongoing physical or psychological problems.

The Continuum of Care for Addictions Nursing

Prevention

Prevention is an anticipatory process that prepares and supports individuals and systems in the creation and reinforcement of healthy behaviors and lifestyles (SAMHSA, 1994). Primary prevention is the reduction or control of causative factors for addiction, and includes reducing risk factors, increasing protective factors, and participating in health service interventions (Teutsch, 1992).

- A *risk factor* is an attitude, belief, behavior, situation, or action that may put a person, group, organization, or community at risk for experiencing addiction. Risk factors should be assessed including biological and environmental vulnerability. Biological vulnerability includes genetic neurochemical predisposition. Risk factors from the environment include traumatic life events, such as sexual, physical, or emotional abuse, and chronic family stress (Snow, 2000a).

- A *protective factor* is an attitude, belief, situation, or action that protects an individual, group, organization, or community from the effects of addictions (SAMHSA, [CSAP] 1994). Protective factors provide resiliency in preventing the development of substance use disorders and other addictions, so that even if the person has numerous risk factors present, there is a buffer that helps prevents abuse or dependence from developing. Having a caring role model as a child is one of the strongest protective factors in prevention of abuse or dependence, much as effectiveness in work, play, and relationships are protective factors for adults (Snow, 2000a). Other protective factors include faith, spirituality, and religious behavior (Booth & Martin, 1998).

A variety of public policies are aimed at prevention of addictions including:

- Legal sanctions
- Decreasing availability
- Use of warning labels
- Removal of cigarette vending machines from public areas
- Prohibiting smoking in public areas
- Increasing alcohol and cigarette taxes
- Random breath testing of drivers
- Raising the legal drinking age
- Increasing sanctions for using or selling illicit drugs
- Increasing server liability
- Workforce initiatives, such as random drug testing

Combined grassroots level community, federal, and state legislative activities have resulted in funded prevention programs targeting vulnerable populations, such as youth, women, and people of color. The U.S. Substance Abuse and Mental Health Services Administration's (SAMHSA) Center for Substance Abuse Prevention (CSAP) initiatives during the 1990s focused on enhancing prevention strategies via training programs for healthcare providers, including training and development of generalist registered nurses, as well as specialty addictions nurses. The numerous CSAP-funded demonstration projects revealed "best practices" information that nurses can use to prevent addictions in their practices. (Allen, 1996; SAMHSA, 1994). Health services research is needed to measure the effectiveness and cost-effectiveness of prevention strategies, to reduce the demand for future healthcare services, and to assess how effective prevention programs are in populations that use high levels of healthcare services (National Advisory Council on Alcohol Abuse and Alcoholism, 1997). See Appendix A for a more detailed description of specific prevention strategies.

Early Intervention (Brief Interventions)

The use of *brief intervention* (BI) has become increasingly important in the continuum of care, particularly with the healthcare system now a managed care model, with reduced reimbursement policies for addiction. BI provides clinicians with intervention strategies for patients engaging in risk use that can increase positive outcomes and reduce the harmful effects of substance use (Sullivan & Fleming, 1997).

Brief interventions include advising the patient about the effects of drug or alcohol use or other at risk behaviors on health status and linking the behaviors with negative health outcomes. Strategies include reviewing findings with the patient, providing educational information (e.g. brochures, reading materials, videotapes) and counseling (Sullivan & Fleming, 1997). Assessing the patient's stage of behavioral change (i.e., pre-contemplation, contemplation, preparation, action, maintenance, and relapse) and providing interventions appropriate to the stage of change is done in a matter-of-fact, non-judgmental manner (Snow, 2000a; Dyehouse & Sommers, 1998). BI, which is timely, focused, and patient-centered, can quickly engage the patient in a therapeutic relationship that promotes behavioral change. Motivating the patient to decide to reduce or eliminate behaviors that demonstrate at risk, or mild to moderate problem use/abuse is referred to as "early intervention." See Appendix B for further discussion of motivational interventions.

Treatment

The Principles of Drug Addiction Treatment (NIDA, 1999) can apply to all addictions. The thirteen principles of *effective* treatment are:

1. No single treatment is appropriate for all persons.

2. Treatment needs to be readily available.

3. Effective treatment attends to multiple needs of the individual.

4. An individual's treatment and services plan must be assessed continually and modified as necessary to ensure that the plan meets the person's changing needs.

5. Remaining in treatment for an adequate period is critical for treatment effectiveness.

6. Counseling (individual or group) and other behavioral therapies are critical components of effective treatment for addiction.

7. Medications are an important element of treatment for many patients, especially when combined with counseling and other behavioral therapies.

8. Addicted individuals with coexisting mental disorders should have both disorders treated in an integrated way.

9. Medical detoxification is only the first stage of addiction treatment and by itself does little to change long-term drug use.

10. Treatment does not need to be voluntary to be effective.

11. Possible lapses into the addictive behavior during the time of treatment must be monitored continuously.

12. Treatment programs should provide assessment for HIV/AIDS, hepatitis B and C, tuberculosis, and other infectious diseases, as well as counseling to help patients modify behaviors that place themselves or others at risk of infection.

13. Recovery from drug addiction can be a long-term process and frequently requires multiple episodes of treatment.

Treatment for addiction and addictive behaviors can be delivered in many different settings. Patients who are participating in treatment for their addictive behaviors are usually in the dependence/addiction stage of the process of addiction. Specialized treatment facilities provide detoxification, counseling, behavioral therapy, medication therapy, case management, and other services from a comprehensive, holistic perspective. These facilities are usually part of local, state, or federal governments and provide detoxification, short-term, residential, or long-term treatment. Treatment can also occur in mental health facilities, clinics, outpatient settings, patient homes, halfway houses, and community-based facilities. Since high rates of other psychiatric disorders co-occur with addiction, many treatment facilities offer dual diagnosis or MISA (mental illness/substance abuse) programs that integrate treatment of co-occurring disorders, such as bipolar disorder, schizophrenia, major depressive disorder, and anxiety disorders with the treatment of a substance use disorder.

Some treatment approaches are specific to setting, but for the most part a variety of therapeutic services and interventions (both behavioral and pharmacological) can be provided in any given setting.

- Cognitive behavioral therapy, motivational interviewing, and brief solution therapy are treatment modalities offered in most treatment programs. Most therapies are offered in groups.

- Exercise, leisure time activities, and stress management are also important components in comprehensive treatment.

- Treatment may also include complementary therapies, such as acupuncture treatment for detoxification, relaxation and imagery, nutritional supplements and antioxidants, and yoga.

- Pharmacological management is used for detoxification, to decrease craving, to manage symptoms associated with withdrawal, for aversion behavioral therapy (e.g. disulfiram), and for treating co-occurring disorders such as bipolar disorder, major depressive disorder, panic disorder and other anxiety disorders, and schizophrenia.

Most treatment programs collaborate with self-help community programs. Self-help is not "treatment" per se, but is most often considered to be an integral aspect of recovery. Self-help groups can complement and extend the effects of professional treatment. The most prominent self-help groups are those affiliated with Alcoholics Anonymous (AA), Narcotics Anonymous (NA), Cocaine Anonymous (CA), Overeaters Anonymous (OA), Sex Anonymous (SA), Gamblers Anonymous (GA), etc. They are all based on the 12-step model. Most patients are encouraged to identify and participate in self-help programs early in intervention and treatment.

Recovery and Relapse Prevention

Persons in the recovery and relapse prevention stage of the process of addiction are often involved in a self-help program or other community support groups (e.g. AA, NA). Self-help and support programs also exist for family members and significant others of patients who are addicted (e.g. AlAnon, NarAnon, and GamAnon). Knowledge about self-help programs increases the ability of nurses to provide adequate support for patients and families with an addiction.

Recovery is enhanced by a focus on lifestyle changes, resolution of grief, family of origin issues, parenting concerns, developmental stages, self management skills, management of symptoms of mental illness such as depression and anxiety, treatment of physical illness, legal and financial stressors, and spiritual health. Ongoing care is critical to recovery and includes an interdisciplinary team to support the patient in the process of recovery.

Persons in the recovery and relapse prevention stage are at risk for relapse at any time. A full-sustained remission for drug and alcohol abuse or dependence is considered to be 12 months without having met any criteria (APA, 2000). Craving may be a strong factor that contributes to the risks for relapse for any addiction. The nurse's role is crucial, including motivating and encouraging the patient during recovery, monitoring for risk factors and symptoms, and intervening early if there is a re-occurrence of symptoms.

Description of Addictions Nursing

Addictions nursing is a distinct specialty practice that integrates biological, behavioral, environmental, psychological, social, and spiritual aspects of human responses to the illness of addiction into the nursing care provided to those affected by this disorder/disease, regardless of the clinical setting. The scope of addictions nursing practice exists on a continuum that ranges from providing care when a problem may not exist (prevention) to providing care when addiction is present.

Addictions nursing practice is knowledge-specific, rather than setting-dependent (Vourakis, 1996), because the potential or actual responses to addictive substances or behaviors manifest themselves in a wide variety of presentations. Wherever nurses practice, they encounter people who are facing issues related to addiction, and must use their knowledge of how addiction develops, the consequences it creates, the processes for preventing the disease or relapses of the disease, and the processes for promoting individual, family, and community health. This knowledge is drawn from the biological, psychological, social, spiritual, and behavioral sciences. Addictions nurses also need a thorough understanding of pathophysiology, neurochemistry, the stages of change in relation to behavior, and the use or overuse of psychological defenses. Addictions nurses need interpersonal skills, critical thinking skills, knowledge of social systems, skill in consultation and collaboration, pharmacology skills, and therapy or counseling skills.

Addictions nurses provide direct care services, but they also consult with other providers, design programs, advocate for clients, and help to shape public policy and access to care. They may choose to specialize their practice to focus on:

- Individuals
- Families
- Communities
- Population or target groups within populations, such as women and children
- Dually diagnosed (MISA) persons with co-occurring disorders (those individuals with two or more DSM-IV diagnoses)
- The elderly
- Specific ethnic or cultural groups

Addictions nurses use knowledge of financing, systems development and change, and awareness of legal and ethical issues to formulate effective policies and procedures. They use evidence-based knowledge to continue to develop and provide state-of-the-art practice. The goal is to provide holistic care that is accessible to all.

Addictions nursing strategies or interventions may be wellness-oriented and focused on health promotion and disease prevention, or they may be illness-oriented and focused on prompt and appropriate treatment of medical conditions associated with addiction. Interventions can also be recovery-oriented with a focus on creating the conditions that foster sobriety, serenity, relapse prevention, and reintegration into effective family, community, school, and work lives.

Phenomena of Concern

Addictions nurses in any clinical setting are concerned with patients with actual or potential responses to addictive substances and behaviors. Because those responses may exist at any point of the wellness–illness continuum, addictions nurses are concerned with:

- Conditions which increase vulnerability to or risk for addiction
- Consequences and impairment that occur when people use those substances or behaviors
- Responses of people to dependence on addictive substances or behaviors
- Conditions that affect recovery and rehabilitation

These responses can be grouped by the following categories, expanded in Table 1 on pages 17–20:

- Physiological effects
- Psychological effects
- Spiritual effects
- Cognitive effects
- Effects on family
- Social/community effects, workplace effects
- Legal effects

TABLE 1. ADDICTIONS PHENOMENA OF CONCERN

Physiological Effects:

(Note: These vary based on the substance used and its pharmacological properties)

- Altered levels of central nervous system responsiveness such as hyperactivity, seizures, and sleep disorders
- Chronic neurological conditions such as neuronal membrane changes, changes in neurochemical processes of the brain, brain cell deterioration, and peripheral nerve deterioration
- Altered psychomotor patterns such as tremors, increased or decreased sensitivity of reflexes
- Alterations of digestive system, including nausea, vomiting, anorexia, nutritional imbalances, chronic gastritis, ulceration of stomach or small intestine, pancreatitis, diarrhea, and constipation
- Alterations in immune system causing increased susceptibility to infections and problems combating infections, such as skin infections, pneumonia, and potential development of HIV infections
- Alterations in cardiovascular system, such as endocarditis, arrhythmias, peripheral vascular disease, alcoholic cardiomyopathy, and hypertension
- Chronic and disabling physical disease processes, including tissue damage, biochemical changes in major organs, and nutritional deficiencies caused by malnutrition, maldigestion, and malabsorption
- Endocrine disorders caused by changes in levels of production of hormones, such as Cushing's syndrome and impotence
- Hepatic disorders, such as fatty liver, hepatitis, and cirrhosis
- Respiratory disorders, including destruction of nasal tissues and structures, upper respiratory infections, emphysema, lung cancer, tuberculosis, and aspiration pneumonia
- Pain syndromes such as neuropathy, decreased response to pain
- Increased risk of transmission of sexually transmitted diseases such as HIV/AIDS, hepatitis C, chlamydia
- Perinatal/neonatal damage, such as fetal alcohol effects, fetal alcohol syndrome, low birth weight, irritability, neuro-developmental delays
- Sleep disorders such as insomnia, nightmares, poor sleep architecture
- Neurochemical or genetic predisposition to developing additional addictions

TABLE 1. ADDICTIONS PHENOMENA OF CONCERN

Psychological Effects:

- Depression, anxiety, shame, anger, denial, conflict within the family, remorse, alienation, fear of discovery, fear of abandonment, loss of control. Chronic tension, irritability, inability to relax without addictive substance or behavior, aggressiveness
- Increased anger and impulse control problems, resulting in family, marital, or other types of violence, physical and mental abuse, suicide ideation and attempts
- Psychiatric disorders and unmanageable feeling states, such as guilt, hopelessness, helplessness, and powerlessness
- Psychosis, paranoia, hallucinations, depersonalization
- Disruption in self-concept; deteriorating sense of self-worth; excessive use of defenses, including denial, rationalization, projection; narrowing of coping skills repertoire
- Learning disabilities, disruptive behaviors, decreased attention in children

Spiritual Effects:

- Disruption in spiritual connectedness
- Diminished purpose in life
- Feelings of meaninglessness
- Loss of control over self
- Powerlessness
- Helplessness
- Hopelessness
- Worthlessness
- Guilt

Cognitive Effects:

- Problems in acquisition of new information, problems in learning new life skills and healthy patterns of living
- Altered states of consciousness, clouded sensorium, delirium
- Impaired problem-solving abilities
- Impaired judgment
- Distorted views of the world and other people
- Disordered thought processes
- Lack of insight into the relationship between addiction and its impact

TABLE 1. ADDICTIONS PHENOMENA OF CONCERN

Effects on Family:

- Family life disruption, crises precipitated by an individual's patterns of addictive behavior
- Altered communication patterns and role performance
- Marital infidelity, nonsupport of dependents
- Enabling and rescuing behaviors, including efforts to assist the person with abuse/ dependency to escape consequences
- Multigenerational dysfunctional patterns of relating and coping that are passed on to later generations.
- Unpredictable behavior at home, financial problems
- Family processes structured around the addiction
- Isolation, lack of maturity
- Attempts to control use
- Inconsistent family structure, rigid roles and rules, closed system
- Co-dependency with poor boundaries, lack of personal control
- Children assuming roles of parents (role reversal)
- Increased use of healthcare resources
- Instability, mistrust
- Effects of addicted family member on children's emotional development
- Giving birth to children with fetal alcohol effects, fetal alcohol syndrome, and neonatal abstinence syndrome

Social/Community Effects:

- Disturbed relationships, altered productivity at work, inability to behave according to socially acceptable norms, deterioration in social life and interactions with friends, spouses, and significant others
- Interference with normal growth and development of individuals, families, and communities
- Increased criminal activity, violence
- Advertising of addictive substances concentrated in vulnerable neighborhoods
- Norms within community which condone use of addictive substances/behaviors
- Transient residents

TABLE 1. ADDICTIONS PHENOMENA OF CONCERN

- Risk factors such as poverty, racism, easy access to substances unemployment, lack of housing
- Strained existing resources, problems with access to services
- Homelessness

Workplace Effects:

- Lack of polices and prevention efforts
- Stressful environments which increase vulnerability to use addictive substances or behaviors
- Employee turnover, absenteeism, lateness
- Decreased morale
- On-the-job accidents
- Violence in the workplace
- Costs to society, including lost productivity, destruction of property and lives, excessive personnel hours required to manage problems related to addiction in the workplace
- Inconsistent behavior at work
- Deterioration in work performance

Legal Effects:

- Driving under the influence
- Prostitution
- Arrests for disturbing the peace
- Increased criminal activity
- Illegal drug sales and distribution systems
- Domestic violence and other violence charges
- Court-ordered evaluation and treatment
- Bankruptcy
- Theft, shoplifting
- Underage use

Special Diagnostic Phenomena

Addictions and addictive behaviors can be associated with other diagnostic phenomena that nurses repeatedly confront. These may include: HIV/AIDS; sexually-transmitted diseases; co-occurring primary addictions and psychiatric disorders; hepatitis; tuberculosis; domestic, family, institutional, interpersonal, and community violence; spinal cord and other disabilities; chronic conditions leading to inadequate pain management; and lung, throat, mouth, and other cancers.

Specialty Practice: Generalist Level

Addictions specialty nurses at the generalist level have expertise in prevention, interventions, and treatment for patients, their families, and groups of individuals affected by addiction. Depending on the clinical setting, they address low risk, at risk, problem use/misuse/abuse and dependency/addiction. These nurses possess demonstrated clinical skills within the specialty, exceeding those of a novice in the field, and have completed additional preparation such as enhanced educational preparation through formal classes in addiction, attendance at professional conferences, informal training through hands-on experience, distance learning through correspondence and Internet courses, and time spent in public self-help groups not related to their own support or recovery.

The nurse's expertise is based on the knowledge and clinical skills required to address alterations in all dimensions of the human system (psychological, biological, cognitive, social, and spiritual) affected by addiction. Such skills include counseling, health education, screening and assessment, clinical interventions aimed at reducing the consequences of addiction, and the promotion of self-management.

Generalist level addictions nursing practice is characterized by interventions that promote and foster health, assess abuse/dependency, assist patients and families to regain or improve their coping mechanisms, and prevent relapse. The nurse should be skilled in developing a therapeutic relationship with patients to foster collaboration in implementation of the plan of care. The patient may be an individual, a family or network of significant others, a group of individuals, or a community.

The following skills and knowledge are foundational for the practice of addictions nursing at the generalist level:

- Theoretical and clinical knowledge at the generalist level of nursing education
- Knowledge and skills in comprehensive nursing assessment, including interviewing, taking a health history, conducting a physical examination, psychosocial assessment, mental status examination, family assessment, and community assessment
- Knowledge and skills related to the use of screening and assessment tools with specific addictive disorders
- Self-awareness as a basis for enhancing engagement with the patient in a therapeutic relationship
- Knowledge of patterns of addiction and the behavioral and physiological responses that accompany these patterns
- Counseling skills with individuals, groups, and families including:
  a) Formal and informal approaches
  b) Techniques specific to substance use and other addictive disorders
  c) Counseling goals:
     1) Development of therapeutic relationship or alliance
     2) Understanding of the health consequences and risks
     3) Identification of unhealthy coping mechanisms
     4) Motivational interviewing to modify the client's view of self and the world
     5) Identifying stage of change and readiness for change
     6) Promoting healthy constructive thoughts, behaviors, and coping strategies
     7) Positive reinforcement for modification of the patient's family, work, and living environments

When working in a residential, community, or hospital-based setting, the addictions nurse has a pivotal role in the development and maintenance of a therapeutic milieu within the treatment unit or program. The goal is to develop mutual respect with the patient in order to provide guidance, support, and direction as the recovery process begins.

Evaluation of the treatment plan and progress in its implementation are continuous and systematic. Because addictions are illnesses characterized by periods of progress and relapse, progress, or lack of progress, toward identified goals requires periodic assessment of the patient's status. This allows the nurse to assist the patient or family in the reformulation of goals, interventions, or a change in priorities. The patient's participation in setting goals and in implementing the treatment plan is an important part of recovery.

Specialty Practice: Advanced Level

The advanced practice registered nurse in addictions (APRN-A) manages patients with addictions and related health problems using a high level of expertise in the assessment, diagnosis, and management of the complex responses of individuals, families, or communities. As well, the APRN-A plans prevention programs in communities through advocacy and planning skills, and influences health policy. Accordingly, the APRN-A has a master's or doctoral degree with a strong focus in addictions, including co-occurring problems of a psychiatric or medical nature or public health and community focus. In addition, during graduate education the APRN-A has clinical experiences focused on addictions practice and continues ongoing clinical experiences related to addictions following graduation.

In addition to the basic addictions nursing practice skills and knowledge, the APRN in addictions has the preparation and skills, based on their educational experience and practice to:

- Complete comprehensive health assessment including complete history, physical examination when appropriate, and mental status assessment.
- Formulate clinical decisions to manage acute and chronic addictions-related illness.
- Provide direct care that includes screening, assessment, diagnosis, and development of a comprehensive treatment plan.
- Order laboratory and other tests.
- Prescribe medications for: management of intoxication, overdose, withdrawal, craving; substitution therapy; and symptom management for co-occurring psychiatric disorders (for APRN-As with prescriptive authority and educational preparation).
- Prescribe nonpharmacological treatments related to addictions and associated health problems.
- Conduct psychotherapy including individual, couples, group, or family.

- Implement health promotion and disease prevention interventions related to addictions.

- Include relevant teaching plans.

- Make accurate referrals and consultations.

- Evaluate outcomes of interventions.

- Conduct or actively participate in addictions research.

- Serve as leader and mentor.

- Collaborate and function as an integral member of an interdisciplinary team.

Some APRN-As have completed a Clinical Nurse Specialist-focused master's degree program or a primary care or specialty (e.g., Psychiatric Mental Health Nurse Practitioner) master's degree Nurse Practitioner program. Other advanced degrees prepare the addictions nurse to focus more on community assessment, population focused interventions, and research aimed at improving the health of communities.

The APRN in addictions combines case management functions with population-specific nursing knowledge, research competencies, expertise in psychotherapy, and the ability to work with complex and severe addictions problems. In community and primary settings, the APRN in addictions, in a leadership role, analyzes the health needs of both individuals and populations, and designs programs that target at-risk groups and cultural and environmental factors, foster health, and prevent abuse and addiction.

The APRN in addictions frequently provides clinical supervision to assist others to further develop their clinical skills. Consultation to healthcare providers and others regarding quality of care related to addictions issues, e.g. detoxification protocols in a general medical setting, can be a significant part of the role.

Additional Activities of Addictions Nurses

Addictions nursing encompasses both prevention of health problems and promotion of optimal health for the individual and society through education. Nurses, as recognized authorities on health, can educate individuals, groups, and communities about risk and protective factors, as well as characteristics of addictive substances. Nurses may integrate experiential learning opportunities to help the learner develop understanding of abuse and addictions and the skills to learn to cope with them.

Health teaching includes communicating about healthy behaviors and relationships, harm reduction strategies, as well as dysfunctional interpersonal and familial patterns, such as codependency and dysfunctional parenting. The nurse works with patients in their activities of daily living to promote adherence to an appropriate health regimen aimed at abstinence from mood altering chemicals, interruption in the compulsive behavior patterns, and effective interaction patterns with significant others.

Case management is a clinical component of the addictions nurse's role in both inpatient and outpatient settings. Nurse case managers employ culturally relevant interventions designed to support the patient's highest level of functioning, enhanced recovery, and progress toward optimal health. The case manager identifies and coordinates various other health and human services as resources for care.

A particularly important role of the addictions nurse is that of advocate, for the purpose of influencing policy. The nursing profession supports each person's right to health care, regardless of social or economic status, personal attributes, or the nature of the person's health problems. Addictions nurses have long fought the battle to help society understand the disease concept of addiction and recognize that addictions treatment works. Their work in state and federal organizations has resulted in increased funding for treatment agencies and research.

Addictions nurses are joining professional or consumer groups to abolish the stigma attached to addictions and to achieve parity between addictions, mental health, and physical illness insurance benefits. These nurses not only support legislation and community action, but also use their professional and political skills to promote the expansion of the healthcare system to address problems of abuse and addiction (e.g. issues of access to care).

In clinical practice, the addictions nurse advocates for the rights of patients. Because of a strong commitment to the health, welfare, and safety of the patient, nurses must be aware of any activity which places the rights or well-being of the patient in jeopardy and take appropriate action on the patient's behalf. It is imperative that addictions nurses working in the community in a variety of settings (public health, free clinic, homeless shelter, methadone clinic) be aware of all the community resources available to the patient and assist the patient in accessing these services. Involvement with community planning boards, advisory groups, paraprofessionals and other key people is an important means by which nurses can mobilize the community's resources and bring about changes that address abuse and addictions needs of particular population groups (adolescents, women, elderly, etc.). See Appendix C for the Code of Ethics for Addictions Nurses, which guides addictions nurses in their practice.

Education for Addictions Nursing Practice

Educational preparation for addictions nursing practice has lagged behind education for other nursing specialties. Federal initiatives have attempted to address this lack of attention to one of the nation's major health problems. The National Institute on Alcohol Abuse and Alcoholism (NIAAA), the National Institute on Drug Abuse (NIDA), and the Office for Substance Abuse Prevention (now the Center for Substance Abuse Prevention) have supported curriculum and faculty development in schools of nursing over the past two decades. As a result of these curriculum grants, several model curricula designed to incorporate addiction information into nursing education at the undergraduate and graduate levels are available for use in undergraduate and graduate nursing programs (Burns, Thompson & Ciccone, 1991; McRee, Babor & Church, 1991; Naegle & D'Arcangelo, 1991).

The generally held public belief that addiction is a moral issue associated with poor judgment, poor impulse control, bad behavior, and an unwillingness to quit using has been the beliefs of some nurses. Research findings support the need for inclusion of addictions content in both undergraduate and graduate nursing curricula. A possible reason for nurses' negative attitudes and false beliefs about addictions has been the lack of evidence-based content about addictions in the nursing curriculum (Starkey, 1980; Smith, 1992; Happell & Taylor, 1999). Inclusion of essential content based on current research and best practices will result in nursing students acquiring the basic skills related to the care of persons with addictions and remove the stigma often associated with addictions (Reisman and Schrader, 1984; Tamlyn 1989; Martinez and Murphy-Parker, 2003). This will in turn affect the quality of care a nurse gives to the addicted client. Several models of curriculum content in addictions have been suggested.

Presently in nursing education much of the emphasis on addictions is related to patients who are currently experiencing addiction and in treatment. Suggested models for curriculum content in addictions include adding a focus on prevention and early intervention strategies, to help nursing students learn the importance of their role in helping prevent substance use disorders and other addictions. Additional suggested content in addictions includes teaching students the neuroanatomy and neurochemistry associated with addiction (Snow, 2000b), assessment for the early signs of at-risk use, brief intervention skills, assessment of withdrawal symptoms, and harm reduction principles. Additional coursework in the pharmacology of addictive substances, the process of addiction, the seductive capabilities of abused substances, and the components of a healthy lifestyle has been suggested. (National Nurses Society on Addictions, 1993)

Other models of curriculum in nursing education related to addictions have been suggested. Recommended content includes the etiology of abuse and dependence, the consequences associated with abuse, the care of affected family members and others surrounding the person relying on addictive substances or behaviors, methods for mobilizing community efforts, treatment and self-help, and the prevention of addiction among healthcare professionals. Addictions content ideally should be integrated throughout nursing curricula, since issues related to addiction occur at all stages of health and disease. It is also recommended that schools of nursing consider development of a policy which offers support for nursing students when they themselves, or a close family member or friend, are experiencing problems with addictions (Murphy-Parker, Knonenbitter & Knonenbitter, 2003; NNSA, 1993; Sullivan, 1995) In addition, undergraduate students need clinical experiences with clients who have addictions-related problems.

Graduate education for specialty practice in addictions nursing should include comprehensive theoretical and research-based content on addictions and development of clinical skills, including screening, comprehensive assessment, differential diagnosis, interventions directed at individuals, families, and communities, and strategies for prevention and rehabilitation. Their clinical practice will include assessment and intervention in various environments that are culture-specific, such as homeless shelters and community centers, as well as office practices, outpatient and hospital settings, home care, and outpatient detoxification. Advanced practice nurses working in other specialty areas should be adequately prepared to screen and assess patients with addictions and refer them to specialty care as needed.

In addition to providing model curricula, federal grants have prepared a cadre of faculty with expertise in alcohol and other drug-related disorders. These faculty serve as resources in their schools, assist in incorporating and implementing addictions content into the curriculum, teach addictions nursing courses, and publish articles about their activities, contributing to the body of knowledge about current and future addictions nursing practice (Gerace, Sullivan, Murphy & Cotter, 1992; Hagemaster, Plumlee, Connors, & Sullivan, 1994; Marcus, Gerace & Sullivan, 1996; 1996, Marcus, 1997).

Certification

A nurse who has the designation of "addictions nurse" meets the specialty's standards of knowledge and experience through certification as a Certified Addictions Registered Nurse (CARN). The CARN has met the qualifications in experience, education, and testing to be recognized in the specialty of addictions nursing at the generalist level. This certification has been offered by the Addictions Nursing Certification Board of the International Nurses Society on Addictions since 1989.

The advanced practice certification for addictions nurses (Certified Addictions Registered Nurse-Advanced Practice, CARN-AP) was first offered by the Addictions Nursing Certification Board of the International Nurses Society on Addictions in 2000. It is based on a national job analysis of the role of the advanced practice nurse in addictions. Criteria for achieving this certification include a master's degree with a specified number of documented hours in advanced practice addictions nursing and a passing score on the certification exam.

Certified Addictions Registered Nurses—CARN and CARN-AP—care for individuals across the life span, their families, and with entire populations. These certified nurses have the potential to reduce the harm to individuals and society related to the use of alcohol, tobacco, and other drugs, and other addictions such as gambling (Finnell, 2002).

Implications for Research

Scientific advances in the specialty of addictions have proliferated in the past few years. Current neurobiological researchers have focused on how addictive substances affect the central nervous system, including the role of neurotransmitters and receptor sites for opiates, alcohol, benzodiazepines, and other substances. Researchers concerned with treatment outcomes have provided evidence to support best practices in relation to treatment for addictions based on specific patient characteristics. Genetic researchers are identifying specific genes involved in addiction, and family pedigree studies hold promise for prevention and early treatment. Transcultural researchers have provided insight into addictions related to specific groups and populations.

Nursing research in addictions is currently contributing to knowledge related to the etiology, prevention, and treatment of addiction. Federally funded faculty development grants have helped ameliorate this deficit, but scientific evidence on the nursing care of persons with addiction disorders needs further research. Recent funding of nurse scientists to conduct alcohol and other drug research through the National Institute on Alcohol Abuse and Alcoholism and the National Institute on Drug Abuse at the National Institutes of Health will help build the nursing science in addictions. Research in addictions nursing is crucial in leading the search for scientifically tested, appropriate, and effective interventions (Compton, 1996). In particular, nurse researchers are needed who will provide the evidence to support nursing interventions aimed at prevention and treatment of addictive disorders related to individuals, families, groups, and communities.

In addition, more research is needed in relation to other forms of addiction, including those classified as addictive behaviors. Nurse scientists are needed who will study all aspects of such addictions as gambling, eating disorders, and sexual addictions. Finally, nurses must disseminate their research findings and build new evidence-based models of treatment. *Journal of Addictions Nursing* provides a vehicle for addictions nurse researchers as well as other addictions researchers to communicate their findings. To meet this objective, additional nurse scientists interested in addictions nursing are needed in doctoral programs. This will increase the total number of addictions nurse researchers available as principal investigators, project directors, educators, and authors of research-based journal articles. Multiple sources of financial support for doctoral education and for research studies must be identified in order for this strategy to be successful.

Nurses must use research-validated and scientific approaches to addictions prevention and treatment. All nurses, including addictions nurses, need to understand evidence-based practice and make that concept a routine part of professional practice.

Peer Assistance

Nurses are vulnerable to the disease of addiction as are other healthcare professionals. Trinkoff, Eaton & Anthony (1991) reported that 17% of nurses reported heavy alcohol use and 3.8% reported illicit drug use. The nurse's license is subject to revocation if there are impaired practice violations related to addictions or other serious psychiatric disorders. Also, patients may suffer harm from the nurse's impaired behavior. Yet nurses with dependence/addiction, like other persons with dependence/addiction, continue to abuse drugs and alcohol despite the risk of major consequences. Interventions are often done by peers to encourage and motivate the nurse to seek help. Nurses have an ethical obligation to advocate for their colleagues who manifest impaired practice and motivate them to seek help through their state peer assistance program, if available. If there is not a peer assistance program then the nurse must be referred to the State Board of Nursing and disciplinary action may ensue.

Peer assistance programs that are alternative to discipline programs are offered in most states to provide monitoring, counseling and case management so that the nurse who is willing to seek help and recovery from the addiction or mental disorder does not face disciplinary action with the State Board of Nursing. Nurses continue in the program in most states for two years, during which time they return to work with some restrictions on their practice (e.g. not being able to work extra shifts).

Nursing organizations, such as the International Nurses Society on Addictions, advocate for all nurses who need help for addictions or other psychiatric disorders to have the opportunity to participate in alternatives to discipline programs, and assist them in establishing return-to-work agreements. A national effort is underway to ensure that all states offer such programs. In 2002 the American Nurses Association passed an update of the 1980 ground-breaking resolution calling for all states to create non-disciplinary programs. The National Student Nurses Association (NSNA) also passed a resolution in 2002 calling for all schools of nursing to implement policies to support nursing students with addictions (Murphy-Parker, Kronenbitter & Kronenbitter, 2003).

Standards of Care for Addictions Nursing

Standard 1. Assessment

The addictions nurse collects patient health data.

Measurement Criteria

1. The addictions nurse determines the priority of data collection according to the patient's immediate health needs.

2. Assessment is individualized based on the patient's age, culture, and medical and biopsychosocial needs.

3. The data are collected in a systematic and ongoing manner, including the following:

Subjective data:

- Chief complaint, symptoms, or focus of concern
- Physical, developmental, cognitive, mental, and emotional health status
- Current and past medications, including prescribed, over the counter, herbal
- Past medical, psychiatric, and addictions history
- Family history including addictions, psychiatric disorders, other health concerns
- Family, community, culture, race, ethnicity systems
- Spiritual health
- Personal, developmental, abuse, and social history
- Work or school adjustment
- Interpersonal relationships, communication skills, and coping patterns
- Current use of psychoactive substances and compulsive behaviors

Objective data:

- Physical health measurements
- Screening, diagnostic and lab measurements
- Mental status examination
- Safety, health promotion and functional assessment
- Strengths and assets that can be used to promote health

4. Assessment is done collaboratively with interdisciplinary team members.

5. Assessment actively includes the patient, family, other healthcare workers, social network, and past and current medical records when appropriate.

6. Data records are synthesized, prioritized, and documented in retrievable form.

7. Assessment techniques are based on clinical judgment and addictions research.

8. Patient data are collected using reliable and valid addictions-specific instruments.

STANDARD 2. DIAGNOSIS

The addictions nurse analyzes the assessment data in determining diagnoses.

Measurement Criteria

1. Diagnoses and potential problem statements are derived from assessment data.

2. Interpersonal, systemic, or environmental circumstances that affect the well-being of the individual, family, or community are identified.

3. The diagnoses are based on an accepted framework that supports the addictions nursing knowledge and judgment used in analyzing the data.

4. Diagnoses are consistent with accepted classifications systems, such as North American Nursing Diagnosis Association (NANDA) *Nursing Diagnosis Classification, International Classification of Diseases* (WHO 1993), and *The Diagnostic and Statistical Manual of Mental Disorders IV-TR* (APA 2001) used in the practice setting.

5. Diagnoses and risk factors are validated with the patient, significant others, family members or guardians, and other healthcare providers when appropriate and possible.

6. Diagnoses identify actual or potential responses to addictive substances/behaviors and health problems of the patient pertaining to:

    •   Maintenance of optimal health and well-being and the prevention of illness.

    •   Self-care limitations or impaired functioning related to psychological and emotional distress.

    •   Deficits in the functioning of significant biological, psychological, spiritual, and cognitive systems.

    •   Emotional stress or crisis components of illness, pain, and disability.

    •   Self-concept changes, developmental issues, and life process changes.

    •   Problems related to emotions such as anxiety, aggression, sadness, loneliness, and grief.

    •   Physical symptoms that occur along with altered psychological functioning.

    •   Alterations in thinking, perceiving, symbolizing, communicating, and decision-making.

- Difficulties in relating to others.

- Behaviors and mental status that indicate the patient is a danger to self or others or has a severe disability.

- Interpersonal, systemic, sociocultural, spiritual, or environmental circumstances or events, which have an effect on the psychological and emotional well-being of the individual, family, or community.

- Symptom management, side effects or toxicity associated with detoxification, psychopharmacologic intervention, and other aspects of the treatment regimen.

- Symptom management related to medical illness.

7. Diagnoses and clinical impressions are documented in a manner that facilitates the identification of patient outcomes and their use in the plan of care.

STANDARD 3. OUTCOME IDENTIFICATION

The addictions nurse identifies expected outcomes individualized to the patient.

Measurement Criteria

Expected outcomes:

1. Are derived from the diagnoses.

2. Are patient-oriented, evidence-based, therapeutically sound, realistic, attainable, and cost effective.

3. Are documented as measurable goals.

4. Are formulated by the nurse and the patient, significant others, and interdisciplinary team members, when possible.

5. Are age-related, culturally appropriate and sensitive, and gender-specific, as well as realistic in relation to the patient's present and potential capabilities and quality of life.

6. Reflect considerations of the associated benefits and costs.

7. Estimate a time for attainment.

8. Provide direction for continuity of care.

9. Serve as a record of change in the patient's health status.

10. Reflect consideration of the patient's bio-psycho-socio-spiritual and cultural needs.

11. Are attainable in relation to resources available to the patient.

12. Are used in comparative data and benchmarking reports with like programs and facilities.

13. Are modified based on changes in the patient's health status.

14. Reflect current scientific knowledge in addictions care.

STANDARD 4. PLANNING

The addictions nurse develops an individualized plan of care that prescribes interventions to attain expected outcomes.

Measurement Criteria

The plan of care:

1. Is developed through collaborative efforts of the addictions nurse, the interdisciplinary treatment team, the patient, and significant others.

2. Uses the nursing process in developing and revising the plan of care.

3. Identifies priorities of care in relation to expected outcomes.

4. States realistic goals in behavioral or measurable terms with expected dates of accomplishment.

5. Incorporates psychotherapeutic and neurobiological theories and principles.

6. Specifies evidence-based interventions that reflect current best practices in addictions nursing.

7. Specifies appropriate interventions, individualized according to the patient's age, gender, developmental stage, ethnicity, and sexual orientation.

8. Includes an educational plan related to the patient's health problems, treatment plan, relapse prevention, self-care, and quality of life issues.

9. Provides the appropriate consultation, referral, and case management to ensure continuity of care.

10. Includes a plan for ongoing treatment of healthcare needs.

11. Is documented in a format that allows modification, interdisciplinary access, and retrieval of data for analysis and research when appropriate.

12. Includes strategies for health promotion, disease prevention, and restoration of health.

13. Reflects current best practices in addictions nursing practice (prevention, intervention, treatment, relapse prevention).

STANDARD 5. IMPLEMENTATION

The addictions nurse implements the interventions identified in the plan of care.

Measurement Criteria

Interventions are:

1.   Implemented within the established plan of care and address identified actual or potential needs of the patient.

2.   Implemented in a safe, timely, ethical, and appropriate manner.

3.   Documented in a format that is related to patient outcomes, accessible to the interdisciplinary team, and retrievable.

4.   Based on current scientific and theoretical knowledge.

5.   Performed according to the nurse's level of education and practice.

STANDARD 5A. THERAPEUTIC ALLIANCE

The addictions nurse uses the "therapeutic self" to establish a therapeutic alliance with the patient and to structure nursing interventions to promote development of insight, coping skills, and motivation for change in behavior that promotes health.

Measurement Criteria

1.   The nurse documents the presence or absence of behavior change that reflect increased knowledge and motivation for change regarding patterns of use, abuse, and dependence related to addictive substances or behaviors.

2.   The nurse documents the degree to which relational skills and health promotion behaviors have been incorporated into the patient's lifestyle.

3.   The relationship established between nurse and patient remains within professional and ethical boundaries.

STANDARD 5B. HEALTH TEACHING

The addictions nurse, through health teaching, assists individuals, families, groups, and communities in achieving satisfying, productive, and healthy patterns of living.

Measurement Criteria

1. Health teaching occurs in the individual, family, group, and community contexts and includes:

    •   Health promotion.

    •   Risk and protective factors

    •   Methods for strengthening resiliency

    •   Patterns of problem use, abuse and addiction

    •   Spiritual, biological, psychosocial, and cognitive components of addiction, and their impact on self, family, and community.

    •   Treatments and their effects on daily living

    •   The process of recovery and relapse prevention

    •   Physical health

    •   Social skills

    •   Developmental, gender, and cultural needs

    •   Parenting and strengthening family coping

2. Educational activities and the learning responses of the individual, family, group, and community are documented.

3. Health teaching methods and strategies are appropriate to the developmental level, learning needs, readiness and ability to learn, health status, education, and culture of the individual, family, group, and community.

STANDARD 5C. SELF-CARE AND SELF-MANAGEMENT

The addictions nurse uses the knowledge and philosophy of self-care and self-management to assist the patient in learning new ways to address stress, maintain self-control, accept personal responsibility, and integrate healthy coping behaviors into life-style choices.

Measurement Criteria

1. The self-care and self-management activities chosen are appropriate to the patient's physical and mental status as well as age, developmental level, gender, ethnicity, and education.

2. The self-care and self-management interventions assist the patient in accepting responsibility for health, including accessing available community support systems such as self-help groups, making personal lifestyle changes, setting realistic goals for behavioral change, and monitoring progress.

3. The self-care and self-management interventions extend to the family and significant others when appropriate to facilitate system change, including accessing community support systems.

4. The nurse documents the level of the patient's ability to respond to involvement in self-help or other support groups as appropriate.

STANDARD 5D. PHARMACOLOGICAL, BIOLOGICAL, AND COMPLEMENTARY THERAPIES

The addictions nurse applies knowledge of pharmacological, biological, and complementary therapies and uses clinical skills to restore the patient's health and prevent consequences from addiction.

Measurement Criteria

The addictions nurse:

1. Uses current research findings and best practices to guide nursing actions related to pharmacology, other biological therapies, and complementary therapies.

2. Monitors pharmacological agents' intended actions, untoward or interactive effects, and therapeutic doses as well as blood levels, vital signs, and laboratory values where appropriate.

3. Directs nursing interventions towards alleviating untoward effects of pharmacological, biological, and complementary therapies.

4. Uses knowledge of signs and symptoms of substance overdose, withdrawal syndrome, and multiple drug-use patterns to promote safety in treatment.

5. Uses knowledge of the appropriate pharmacological and other biological treatments of psychiatric and medical problems that commonly coexist with addictions in monitoring the patient's care.

6. Educates the patient and family of the potential for abuse of selected pharmacological agents.

7. Evaluates the patient's response to the administered medications and therapies and documents the response.

8. Communicates observations about the patient's response to pharmacological, biological, and complementary interventions to other healthcare providers when appropriate.

9. Teaches the patient the beneficial effects and potential adverse effects of prescribed medications, biological treatment, and complementary therapies.

10. Provides the patient information regarding costs of using pharmacological, biological, and complementary therapies in making informed choices.

STANDARD 5E. THERAPEUTIC MILIEU

The addictions nurse structures, provides, and maintains a therapeutic environment in collaboration with the patient and other healthcare providers.

Measurement Criteria

1. The patient is familiarized with the physical environment, the schedule of groups and activities, rights and responsibilities, the rules and regulations that govern behavior, and the goals of the treatment team.

2. Current knowledge and best practices of the effects of environment on the patient are used to promote a safe, therapeutic environment.

3. The therapeutic environment is designed in accordance with accreditation standards, utilizing the physical environment, social structure, culture, and other available resources.

4. Therapeutic communication among patients and staff supports an effective milieu.

5. Specific activities are selected that meet the patient's physical, spiritual, psychological, and behavioral health needs.

6. Limits of any kind (e.g., restriction of privileges) are the least restrictive necessary, maintain the dignity of the patient, and are used only to ensure the safety of the patient and others.

7. The patient is given information about the need for limits and the conditions necessary for removal of the restriction, as appropriate.

8. Patient orientation to, participation in, and response to the therapeutic milieu are documented.

STANDARD 5F. COUNSELING

The addictions nurse uses counseling interventions to assist patients in promoting healthy coping abilities, preventing addiction, and addressing issues related to patterns of abuse and addiction.

Measurement Criteria

1. Counseling interventions include interdisciplinary and peer collaboration to plan and facilitate achievement of counseling goals.

2. The patient is included in the planning, goal setting, and evaluation of outcomes.

3. Counseling interventions are documented on the treatment plan and medical record.

4. Confidentiality issues are managed with ethical integrity and according to federal, state, and professional confidentiality guidelines.

5. Referral sources for additional therapy, psycho-education programs (e.g. parenting classes), and self-help groups are provided to the patient and family as appropriate.

6. Counseling strategies are used to engage the patient, family, and significant others in the therapeutic process to promote improved relationships and behavioral change.

7. The addictions nurse participates in individual and group counseling within parameters of certification, state, and employer expectations

STANDARD 6. EVALUATION

The addictions nurse evaluates the patient's progress toward attainment of expected outcomes.

Measurement Criteria

1. Evaluation is systematic, ongoing, and outcome-based.

2. The patient, significant others, and healthcare providers are involved in the evaluation process, when appropriate.

3. The patient's responses to interventions are documented in a format related to expected outcomes and easily accessible to the interdisciplinary team.

4. Ongoing assessment data are used to revise diagnoses, outcomes, and the plan of care as needed.

STANDARDS OF PROFESSIONAL PERFORMANCE

STANDARD 7. QUALITY OF CARE

The addictions nurse systematically evaluates the quality of care and effectiveness of nursing practice.

Measurement Criteria

The addictions nurse:

1. Participates in outcomes-based quality improvement activities as appropriate to the nurse's position, education, and practice environment. Such activities may include:

   - Identification of aspects of care important for quality monitoring (e.g., Functional status, symptom management, safety, patient satisfaction, and quality of life)

   - Analysis of quality of care data to identify opportunities for improving care

   - Development of policies, procedures, and practice guidelines to improve quality of care

   - Identification of indicators used to monitor quality of care and effectiveness of nursing care

   - Collection of data to monitor quality of care and effectiveness of nursing care

   - Formulation of recommendations to improve nursing practice or patient outcomes

   - Implementation of activities to enhance the quality of nursing practice

   - Participation on interdisciplinary teams that evaluate clinical practice or health services

2. Uses the results of outcomes-based quality improvement activities to initiate changes in addictions nursing practice.

3. Uses the results of outcomes-based quality improvement activities to initiate changes throughout the healthcare delivery system, as appropriate.

STANDARD 8. PERFORMANCE APPRAISAL

The addictions nurse evaluates their own nursing practice in relation to professional practice standards and relevant statutes and regulations.

Measurement Criteria

The addictions nurse:

1. Engages in performance appraisal of their own clinical practice and role performance with peers or supervisors on a regular basis, identifying areas of strength as well as areas for professional and practice development.

2. Seeks constructive feedback regarding practice and role performance from peers, professional colleagues, patients, and others.

3. Takes action to achieve goals identified during performance appraisal and peer review, resulting in changes in practice and role performance.

4. Engages in a performance improvement plan seeking to achieve identified performance improvement measures related to job performance.

5. Participates in peer review activities as appropriate.

6. Self-evaluates practice based on patient outcomes and current research findings.

7. Changes practice based on knowledge of current professional practice standards, laws, and regulations.

STANDARD 9. EDUCATION

The addictions nurse acquires and maintains current knowledge and competency in nursing practice.

Measurement Criteria

The addictions nurse:

1. Participates in ongoing professional educational activities to improve clinical knowledge, enhance role performance, and increase knowledge of professional issues.

2. Seeks experience and independent learning activities that reflect current research-based clinical practice, in order to maintain and further develop clinical skills and competency.

3. Seeks additional knowledge and skills appropriate to the specialty area and practice setting by participating in educational programs and activities, conferences, workshops, and interdisciplinary professional meetings.

4. Documents their educational activities.

5. Achieves and maintains professional certification.

6. Bases practice in current scientific and theoretical knowledge and research findings.

STANDARD 10. COLLEGIALITY

The addictions nurse interacts with and contributes to the professional development of peers, and treats other healthcare providers as colleagues.

Measurement Criteria

The addictions nurse:

1. Uses opportunities in practice to exchange knowledge, skills, and clinical observations with colleagues and others.

2. Assists others in identifying teaching or learning needs related to clinical cases, role performance, and professional development.

3. Provides peers with constructive feedback regarding their practice.

4. Contributes to an environment that is conducive to the clinical education of nursing students, other healthcare students, and employees as appropriate.

5. Actively promotes interdisciplinary collaboration to enhance professional practice.

6. Contributes to a supportive and healthy work environment.

7. Participates in local, state, national, and international professional associations to address addiction.

STANDARD 11. ETHICS

The addictions nurse's decisions and actions on behalf of patients are determined and implemented in an ethical manner.

Measurement Criteria

The addictions nurse:

1. Observes and maintains patient confidentiality within legal and regulatory parameters.

2. Uses *Code of Ethics for Nurses With Interpretive Statements* (ANA, 2001) and *Code of Ethics for Addictions Nurses* (NNSA, 1996) to guide practice.

3. Follows the ethical responsibilities and principles of conduct prescribed by the facility where they are employed.

4. Informs the patient of the risks, benefits, and expected outcomes of healthcare regimens.

5. Delivers care in a nonjudgmental and nondiscriminatory manner that is sensitive to patient diversity.

6. Delivers care in a manner that preserves patient autonomy, dignity, and rights.

7. Seeks available resources when necessary in formulating ethical decisions.

8. Contributes to resolving the ethical dilemmas or problems of patients and healthcare systems.

9. Acts as a patient advocate and assists patients in developing skills so they can advocate for themselves.

10. Performs interventions in a safe, ethical manner.

STANDARD 12. COLLABORATION

The addictions nurse collaborates with the patient, significant others, and other healthcare providers in providing patient care.

Measurement Criteria

The addictions nurse:

1. Communicates with the patient, significant others, and other healthcare providers regarding patient care.

2. Consults with other healthcare providers regarding patient care as needed.

3. Makes referrals, including provisions for continuity of care, as needed.

4. Collaborates with the patient, family, and other healthcare providers in the formulation of outcomes of care, and in the decisions related to care and the delivery of services.

5. Collaborates with healthcare providers and members of the community to increase the community's capacity to prevent and address addictions.

STANDARD 13. RESEARCH

The addictions nurse uses theory and evidence from research findings to guide practice.

Measurement Criteria

The addictions nurse:

1. Uses interventions substantiated by theory and research, and appropriate to the nurse's position, education, and practice environment, to develop a plan of care.

2. Participates in research activities appropriate to the nurse's position, education, and practice environment. Such activities may include:

   • Identification of clinical or behavioral health problems suitable for nursing research

   • Participation in data collection in research projects

   • Participation in a unit, department, organization, or community research committees or programs

   • Sharing of research activities with others

   • Implementation of research projects in the appropriate setting

   • Critiquing or evaluating research for application to practice

   • Use of research findings in the development of policies, procedures, guidelines, and benchmarks for patient care

3. Disseminates relevant research finding with nurses and other health professionals through presentations, publications, and practice.

STANDARD 14. RESOURCE UTILIZATION

The addictions nurse considers factors related to safety, effectiveness, and cost in planning and delivering patient care.

Measurement Criteria

The addictions nurse:

1. Analyzes factors related to safety, effectiveness, availability, and cost when choosing between practice options that would result in the same expected patient outcome.

2. Assists the patient and significant others in becoming informed consumers about the cost, risks, and benefits of treatment and care.

3. Assists the patient and significant others in identifying and securing appropriate and available services to address health-related needs.

4. Assigns or delegates tasks, as defined by the State Nurse Practice Acts, based on the needs and condition of the patient, and according to the knowledge and skills of the designated caregiver.

5. Participates in ongoing resource utilization review, including facility resources, marketing, and level of treatment needed by each patient.

Advanced Practice Standards of Care for Addictions Nursing

Standard 1. Assessment

The advanced practice addictions registered nurse collects comprehensive patient health data.

Measurement Criteria

The advanced practice addictions registered nurse:

1.   Bases assessment techniques on theory, research, and best practices.

2.   Initiates and interprets diagnostic tests and procedures relevant to the patient's current status as indicated.

Standard 2. Diagnosis

The advanced practice addictions registered nurse critically analyzes the assessment data in determining the diagnoses.

Measurement Criteria

The advanced practice addictions registered nurse:

1.   Derives and prioritizes diagnoses from the assessment data using appropriate complex clinical reasoning.

2.   Formulates a differential diagnosis by systematically analyzing clinical and other related findings.

3.   Makes diagnoses using advanced synthesis of information obtained during the interview, physical examination, mental status exam, diagnostic tests, or diagnostic procedures.

4.   Bases differential diagnoses on criteria consistent with accepted classifications, such as current editions of *The Diagnostic and Statistical Manual of Mental Disorders IV-TR* (2000) and *The International Classification of Diseases 9 and 10* (1993).

STANDARD 3. OUTCOME IDENTIFICATION

The advanced practice registered nurse identifies expected outcomes derived from the assessment data and diagnoses, and individualizes expected outcomes with the patient and the healthcare team when appropriate.

Measurement Criteria

Expected outcomes are:

1. Identified with consideration of the associated risks, benefits, costs, availability and access.

2. Consistent with current theoretical, scientific, and clinical best practices knowledge.

3. Modified based on changes in the patient's healthcare status.

4. Identified with consideration of the entire wellness–illness addictions continuum.

5. Consistent with the patient's age, ethnicity, and socioeconomic and environmental circumstances.

STANDARD 4. PLANNING

The advanced practice addictions registered nurse develops a comprehensive treatment plan that includes interventions to attain expected outcomes.

Measurement Criteria

The comprehensive treatment plan:

1. Describes the assessment and diagnostic strategies and therapeutic interventions that reflect current addictions healthcare knowledge, theory, research, and practice.

2. Reflects the responsibilities of the advanced practice addictions registered nurse and the patient, and may include delegation of responsibilities to others.

3. Addresses strategies for promotion and restoration of health and prevention of illness, injury, and disease through independent clinical decision-making.

4. Is documented and modified to provide direction to other members of the healthcare team.

STANDARD 5. IMPLEMENTATION

The advanced practice addictions registered nurse prescribes, orders, or implements addictions interventions and treatments for the plan of care.

Measurement Criteria

The advanced practice addictions registered nurse:

1. Prescribes, performs, or implements interventions and treatments with knowledge of theory, research findings, and best practices.

2. Performs interventions and treatments within the scope of advanced practice addictions registered nursing.

STANDARD 5A. CASE MANAGEMENT AND COORDINATION OF CARE

The advanced practice addictions registered nurse provides comprehensive clinical coordination of care and case management.

Measurement Criteria

The advanced practice addictions registered nurse:

1. Provides case management and clinical coordination of care services using sophisticated data synthesis with consideration of the patient's complex needs and desired outcomes.

2. Negotiates health-related services and additional specialized care with the patient, appropriate systems, agencies, and providers.

STANDARD 5B. CONSULTATION

The advanced practice addictions registered nurse provides consultation to influence the plan of care for patients, enhance the abilities of others to provide quality care to addicted patients, and effect change in the system.

Measurement Criteria

1. Consultation activities are based on theory, research results, and best practices.

2. Consultation is based on mutual respect and defined role responsibility established with the patient.

3. Consultation recommendations are communicated in terms that facilitate understanding and involve the patient in decision-making.

4. The decision to implement the system change or plan of care remains the responsibility of the patient.

5. The decision to seek consultation is based on the patient's complex needs and the advance practice addictions registered nurse's recognition of need for additional expertise in managing patient care.

STANDARD 5C. HEALTH PROMOTION, HEALTH MAINTENANCE, AND HEALTH TEACHING

The advanced practice addictions registered nurse employs complex strategies, interventions, and teaching to promote, maintain, and improve health and prevent illness and injury.

Measurement Criteria

1. Health promotion and disease, illness, and injury prevention strategies are based on assessment of risks, learning theory, epidemiological principles, and the patient's health beliefs and practices.

2. Health promotion, maintenance, and teaching methods are appropriate to the patient's developmental level, learning needs, readiness and ability to learn, and culture.

STANDARD 5D. PRESCRIPTIVE AUTHORITY AND TREATMENT

The advanced practice addictions registered nurse uses prescriptive authority, procedures, and treatments in accordance with educational preparation, state and federal laws and regulations, applicable nurse practice acts, and appropriate advanced practice certification to treat illness and improve functional health status or to provide preventive care.

Measurement Criteria

The advanced practice addictions registered nurse:

1. Prescribes treatment interventions and procedures according to the patient's healthcare needs, based on current knowledge, practice, theory and research.

2. Performs procedures as needed in the delivery of comprehensive care.

3. Prescribes pharmacologic agents based on sound clinical decision-making using knowledge of pharmacological and physiological principles.

4. Prescribes specific pharmacologic agents or treatments based on clinical indicators or on the patient's status and needs, including the results of diagnostic and laboratory tests, as appropriate.

5. Monitors intended effects and potential adverse effects of pharmacologic and non-pharmacologic treatments, and adjusts them to promote optimal response in the patient.

6. Provides appropriate information about intended effects, potential adverse effects of the proposed prescription, costs, and alternative treatments and procedures to the patient.

STANDARD 5E. PSYCHOTHERAPY AND COMPLEMENTARY THERAPY

The advanced practice addictions registered nurse conducts individual, group, and family psychotherapy, and educates about and evaluates the use of complementary therapies to promote healthy lifestyles, prevent addictive behaviors, treat addictions and improve health status and functional abilities.

Measurement Criteria

1. Therapeutic modalities are individualized for the patient based on current theory, research, and best practices to prevent addiction and promote recovery.

2. Expected outcomes of psychotherapy are mutually determined based on patient need, and modified as necessary as recognized by both the patient and the advanced practice addiction registered nurse.

3. Theory, research, and the practice of complementary therapies are presented to the patient to ensure informed choices.

4. Complementary therapies are used by the advanced practice addictions registered nurse to promote health and well being of the patient, specifically when based on advanced training or certification.

STANDARD 5F. REFERRAL

The advanced practice addictions registered nurse identifies the need for additional care and makes referrals as needed.

Measurement Criteria

1. As a primary provider, the advanced practice addictions registered nurse facilitates continuity of care by implementing recommendations from referral sources.

2. The advanced practice addictions registered nurse refers directly to specific providers for additional care based upon patient needs, with consideration of benefits and costs.

STANDARD 6. EVALUATION

The advanced practice addictions registered nurse evaluates the patient's progress in attaining expected outcomes.

Measurement Criteria

1. The advanced practice addictions registered nurse evaluates the accuracy of diagnoses and effectiveness of interventions in relation to the patient's attainment of the expected outcomes.

2. The evaluation process is based on advanced knowledge, practice, theory and research, and results in revision or resolution of diagnoses, expected outcomes, and plan of care.

ADVANCED PRACTICE STANDARDS OF PROFESSIONAL PERFORMANCE FOR ADDICTIONS NURSING

STANDARD 7. QUALITY OF CARE

The advanced practice addictions registered nurse develops criteria for and evaluates the quality of care and effectiveness of advanced practice addictions registered nurses.

Measurement of Criteria

The advanced practice addictions registered nurse:

1. Assumes a leadership role as a clinical expert in establishing and monitoring standards of practice to improve care for patients with addictions.

2. Uses the results of quality of care activities to initiate changes throughout the healthcare system as appropriate.

3. Participates in efforts to facilitate timely treatment of the patient and minimize costs and unnecessary duplication of testing or other diagnostic activities.

4. Analyzes factors related to safety, satisfaction, effectiveness, and cost/benefit options with the patient, and other providers as appropriate.

5. Analyzes organizational systems for barriers to treatment, and promotes enhancements that affect patient healthcare status.

6. Bases the evaluation of care on current knowledge, practice, and research.

7. Seeks professional advanced practice certification in addictions nursing.

Standard 8. Self-Evaluation

The advanced practice addictions registered nurse continuously evaluates their nursing practice in relation to professional practice standards and relevant statutes and regulations, and is accountable to the public and to the profession for providing competent clinical care.

Measurement Criteria

The advanced practice addictions registered nurse:

1. Has the inherent responsibility as a professional to evaluate their performance according to the standards of the profession, and various regulatory bodies, and to take action to improve practice.

2. Seeks feedback regarding their practice and role performance from peers, professional colleagues, patients, and others.

3. Self-evaluates their practice based on patient outcomes.

Standard 9. Education

The advanced practice addictions registered nurse acquires and maintains current knowledge and skills in addictions practice.

Measurement Criteria

The advanced practice addictions registered nurse:

1. Uses current healthcare research to expand clinical knowledge, enhance role performance, and increase knowledge of professional issues.

2. Seeks experiences and formal and independent learning activities to maintain and develop clinical and professional skills and knowledge.

STANDARD 10. LEADERSHIP

The advanced practice addictions registered nurse serves as a leader and a role model for the professional development of peers, colleagues, and others.

Measurement Criteria

The advanced practice addictions registered nurse:

1. Contributes to the professional development of others to improve patient care and to foster the profession's growth.

2. Brings creativity and innovation to nursing practice to improve care delivery.

3. Participates in professional nursing organization activities.

4. Works to influence policy-making bodies to improve patient care and promote access to care.

STANDARD 11. ETHICS

The advanced practice addictions registered nurse integrates ethical principles and norms in all areas of practice.

Measurement Criteria

The advanced practice addictions registered nurse:

1. Maintains a therapeutic and professional relationship and discusses the delineation of roles and parameters of the relationship with the patient.

2. Informs the patient of the risks, benefits, and outcomes of healthcare regimens.

3. Contributes to resolving the ethical problems or dilemmas of individuals or systems.

Standard 12. Interdisciplinary Process

The advanced practice addictions registered nurse promotes an interdisciplinary process in providing patient care.

Measurement Criteria

The advanced practice addictions registered nurse:

1. Works with other disciplines to enhance patient care via interdisciplinary activities, which may include education, consultation, management, technological development or research opportunities.

2. Facilitates an interdisciplinary process with other members of the healthcare team in implementing the plan of care.

Standard 13. Research

The advanced practice addictions registered nurse utilizes theory and research to discover, examine, and evaluate knowledge, theories, and creative approaches to healthcare practice.

Measurement Criteria

The advanced practice addictions registered nurse:

1. Critically evaluates practice in light of past and current research findings disseminated by the National Institutes of Health (NIAAA and NIDA), professional journals such as *Journal of Addictions Nursing*, and other sources.

2. Identifies relevant research questions in practice related to addiction.

3. Participates in related research as available.

4. Disseminates relevant research findings through practice, education, publication, or consultation.

GLOSSARY

Abuse. A maladaptive pattern of substance use. (See *Substance abuse*.)

Addiction. A complex neurobiobehavioral disorder characterized by impaired control, compulsive use, dependency, and craving for the activity, substance, or food. Relapses are possible even after long periods of abstinence (National Institute on Drug Abuse [NIDA], 2002b; Wilcox & Erickson, 2000). Addiction is often (but not always) accompanied by physiological dependence, consisting of a withdrawal syndrome, or tolerance (NIDA, 2002a). Factors contributing to the development of addiction include genetic predisposition, the reinforcing properties and access to the substance, food or activity, family and peer influences, sociocultural environment, personality, and existing psychiatric disorders (Goldstein, 1994). The terms addictive disorder and addiction are used interchangeably.

At-risk use. The occasional abuse of substances without yet experiencing negative consequences of substance abuse (Adapted from CSAT: SAMHSA, 1997).

Co-occurring disorder. The concurrent presence of two or more independent (but invariably interactive) disorders/conditions, such as substance abuse, physical illness, mental retardation, or mental illness (CSAT: SAMHSA, 1994).

Craving. The conscious awareness of the desire to take a drug. It is a complex neurobiobehavioral phenomenon based on previous experiences with addictive substances or activities (Goldstein, 1994; Ruden and Byalick, 1997; Drummond, 2001).

Dependency. Synonymous with addiction. (See *Addiction; Substance dependence*.)

Detoxification. Preventing or reducing the symptoms of withdrawal from alcohol or other drugs with the goal of "normalization of the person's body chemistry, primarily the neurochemistry, so that the individual is able to function in a manner similar to that experienced prior to the consumption of the substance" (Feigenbaum & Allen, 1996, p. 142).

Eating disorders. Neurobiobehavioral disorders characterized by the inability to regulate eating habits and frequent tendency to overuse or underuse food that interferes with biological, psychological, and sociocultural integrity. Illnesses associated with maladaptive eating regulation responses include anorexia nervosa, bulimia nervosa, and binge eating disorder (Cochrane, 2001, p. 527; American Psychiatric Association [APA], 2000; CSAT: SAMHSA, 1997).

Harm/risk reduction. The "application of methods designed to reduce harm (and risk of harm) associated with ongoing or active addictive behaviors" (Marlatt & Tapert, 1993; Marlatt . & Witkiewitz, 2002).

Impulse-control disorder. Failure to resist an impulse, drive, or temptation to perform an act that is harmful to the person or to others (Blum et al, 1996, Blum et al, 2000; Nestler, 2001; Roberts & Koob, 1997). One example is *pathological gambling* characterized by persistent and recurrent maladaptive gambling behavior that disrupts personal, family, or vocational pursuits (Adapted from APA, 2000, p. 671).

Low risk use. Consumption of small amounts of substances infrequently and not in high-risk situations (Adapted from CSAT: SAMHSA, 1997).

Physiological dependence. A state of adaptation to a substance manifested by tolerance or withdrawal (APA, 2000; NIDA, 2002a).

Prevention. Health care activities aimed at persons who currently do not have the disease or are in the early stages of the disease, rather than the treatment of disease. Prevention activities include reduction of risk, promotion of health behaviors that prevent occurrences of disease and reduce harm (Marlatt & Witkiewitz, 2002), and early detection and treatment to prevent the development of additional consequences of the disease (Ervin, 2002).

Relapse. A recurrence of problem substance use or activity in someone who was abstinent from that substance use or activity (Trachtenberg & Fleming, 1994). It is considered a "normal part of the cycle of change" (Velasquez, Mauer, Crouch & DiClemente, 2001, p. 189) in the recovery from addiction, which involves experiencing a "slip" and reverting to exhibiting the addictive behavior.

Remission. The state in which a person is free of symptoms of substance dependence, substance abuse, impulse disorder, or eating disorder.

Substance abuse. A maladaptive pattern of substance use (i.e., problem use) within the previous 12 months, leading to clinically significant impairment or distress as manifested by repeated occurrence of one or more of the following: (1) failure to fulfill major role obligations, (2) use in physically hazardous situations, (3) legal problems, and (4) continued use despite consequences resulting from use. (Adapted from APA, 2000.)

Substance dependence. A maladaptive substance use pattern within the previous 12 months characterized by three or more of the following symptoms: (1) tolerance, (2) withdrawal, (3) uncontrolled use, persistent desire, or unsuccessful efforts to reduce substance consumption, (4) a great amount of time spent using or recovering from substance use, (5) a reduction in social, occupational, or recreational activities related to use, or (6) continued use despite knowledge of a persistent physical or psychological problem related to the use (Adapted from APA, 2000). *Alcoholism, chemical dependency,* and *substance dependence* are used interchangeably with the term *addiction*.

Substance misuse. The use of a psychoactive substance (drug or alcohol) for the purpose other than that for which it was intended, and that causes physical, social, and psychological harm. The term is also used to represent the pattern of use: experimental, recreational, and dependent (Rassool, 1998 [as cited in Rassool, 2002]).

Substance Use Disorder (SUD). The "spectrum of disorders encompassed in alcohol and/or drug abuse and dependence that are attributed to problematic consumption or illicit use of alcoholic beverages, tobacco products, and drugs, including misuse of prescription drugs." (Haack & Adger, 2002, p.345 modified from U.S.: DHHS 2000). Substance use disorders are on a continuum of increasing severity and impairment of function and include low risk use, at risk use, abuse, and dependence (CSAT/SAMHSA, 1997).

Substances. Psychoactive chemicals, including alcohol, tobacco, and other drugs.

Tolerance. The body's adaptation to the continued presence (Feigenbaum & Allen, 1996, p. 140) of a drug that results in the need for greatly increased amounts of the substance to achieve intoxication (or the desired effect) or a markedly diminished effect with continued use of the same amount of the substance. The degree to which tolerance develops varies greatly across substances (APA, 2000, p. 192).

Withdrawal syndrome. A predictable group of signs and symptoms resulting from abrupt removal of, or a rapid decrease in, the regular dose of a psychoactive substance. The syndrome is often characterized by overactivity of the physiologic functions that were suppressed by the drug or depression of the functions that were stimulated by the drug (NIDA, 2002a).

~~~~

The above definitions are used with permission from Armstrong et al, Core Curriculum for Addictions Nursing (2005). International Nurses Society on Addictions.

REFERENCES

Adlaf, E. M. & Ialomiteanu, A. (2000). Prevalence of problem gambling in adolescents: Findings from the 1999 Ontario student drug use survey. *Canadian Journal of Psychiatry*, 45 (8) 752–755.

Allen, K., ed. (1996). *Nursing Care of the Addicted Client*. Philadelphia: Lippincott.

American Nurses Association (1984). *Addictions and psychological dysfunction in nursing: The profession's response to the problem*. Kansas City, MO: American Nurses Association.

American Nurses Association, National Nurses Society on Addictions, & Drug and Alcohol Nurses Association (1987). *Care of clients with addictions: Dimensions of nursing practice*. Kansas City, MO: American Nurses Association.

American Nurses Association. (1996). *Scope and Standards of Advanced Practice Registered Nursing*. Washington, DC: American Nurses Publishing.

American Nurses Association. (1998). *Scope and Standards of Clinical Nursing Practice, Second Edition*. Washington, DC: American Nurses Publishing.

American Psychiatric Association. (2000) *Diagnostic and statistical manual, 4th ed., text revision*. Washington, DC: American Psychiatric Association.

Armstrong, M., Feigenbaum, J., Savage, C., Snow, D., & Vourakis, C., eds. (2005). *Core curriculum of addictions nursing, 2nd edition*. Raleigh, NC: International Nurses Society on Addiction.

Blum, K., Braverman, E. R., Holder, J. M., Lubar, J. F., Monastra, V. J., Miller, D., Lubar, J. O., Chen, T. J., & Comings, D. E. (2000). Reward deficiency syndrome: A biogenetic model for the diagnosis and treatment of impulsive, addictive, and compulsive behaviors. *Journal of Psychoactive Drugs*, 32 (Supplement), i–iv, 1–112.

Blum, K., Cull, J. G., Braverman, E. R., & Comings, D. E. (1996). Reward deficiency syndrome. *American Scientist*, 84, 132–145.

Blume, S. (1997). Pathological gambling. In *Substance abuse: a comprehensive textbook, 3rd ed.*, Lowinson, J.; Ruiz, P.; Millman, R.; & Langrod, J., 330–337. Baltimore: Williams & Wilkins.

Blundell, J.E. & Hill, A.J. (1993). Binge eating: Psychobiological mechanisms. In *Binge eating—Nature, assessment, and treatment*, Fairburn, C.G. & Wilson, G.T., eds., 206–224. New York: Guilford Press.

Booth, J. & Martin, J.E. (1998). Spiritual and religious factors in substance use, dependence and recovery. In *Handbook of religious & mental health*, Koenig, H.G., ed. 175–200. New York: NY: Academic Press.

Buckner, M. (2002). *Substance abuse among nursing students. Dean's notes: A communication service to nursing school deans, administrators, and faculty.* Anthony J. Jannetti, Inc.

Burns, E., Thompson. ,A. & Ciccone, J. (1991). *An addictions curriculum for nurses and other helping professionals.* Columbus, OH: Ohio State University.

CSAT: SAMHSA (Center for Substance Abuse Treatment. Substance Abuse and Mental Health Service Administration). (1999). *Enhancing motivation for change in substance abuse treatment: Treatment Improvement Protocol (TIP).* Series 35. Washington, DC: Department of Health and Human Services publication No. (SMA) 99-3354.

CSAT/SAHMSA (Center for Substance Abuse Treatment. Substance Abuse and Mental Health Services Administration.) (1997). *A guide to substance abuse services for primary care clinicians: Treatment improvement protocol (TIP).* Series 24. Washington, DC: Department of Health and Human Services publication No. (SMA) 97-3139, 1–23.

CSAT/SAHMSA (Center for Substance Abuse Treatment. Substance Abuse and Mental Health Services Administration.) (1994). *Assessment and treatment of patients with coexisting mental illness and alcohol and other drug abuse. (TIP).* Series 9. Washington, DC: Department of Health and Human Services publication No. (SMA) 94-2078, 3–7.

CSAT/SAHMSA (Center for Substance Abuse Prevention. Substance Abuse and Mental Health Services Administration.) (1994) *Nurse training course: Prevention of alcohol, tobacco, and other drug problems.* Rockville, MD: U.S. Department of Health and Human Services. Substance Abuse and Mental Health Services Administration.

Cochrane, C. E. (2001). Eating regulation responses and eating disorders. In *Principles and practices of psychiatric nursing (7th ed.)*, Stuart, G.W. & Laraia, M.T., eds., 526–547. St. Louis: C. V. Mosby.

Compton, M. (1996). Research in addictions nursing. In *Nursing care of the addicted client,* Allen, K.M., ed., 304–330. Philadelphia: Lippincott.

Davis, C. & Claridge, G. (1998). The eating disorders as addiction: A psychobiological perspective. *Addictive Behaviors*, 23: 463–475.

Drummond, D.C. (2001), Theories of drug craving, ancient and modern. *Addiction,* 96:33–46.

Dyehouse, Janice M. & Sommers, Marilyn Sawyer. (1998). Brief intervention after alcohol-related injuries. *Nursing clinics of North America,* Vol. 33(1): 93–104.

Ervin, N.E. (2002). *Advanced Community Health Nursing Practice.* Saddle River, New Jersey: Prentice Hall.

Feigenbaum, J. C. & Allen, K. M. (1996). Detoxification. In *Nursing care of the addicted client,* Allen, K.M., ed., 139–176. Philadelphia: Lippincott.

Finnell, D. (2002) *Certification in addictions nursing: Promoting and protecting the health of the public.* A white paper. Raleigh, NC: Addictions Nursing Certification Board & International Nurses Society on Addiction.

Gerace, L., Sullivan, E. J., Murphy, S. & Cotter, F. (1992). Faculty development and curriculum change in alcohol and other drug abuse. *Nurse Educator,* 17(1), 24–27.

Gold, M.; Johnson, C.; & Stennie, K. (1997). Eating disorders. In *Substance abuse: A comprehensive textbook, 3rd ed.,* Lowinson, J., Ruiz, P., Millman, R. & Langrod, J., eds., 319–330. Baltimore: Williams & Wilkins.

Goldstein A. (1994). *Addiction: From biology to drug policy.* New York: WH Freeman.

Goodman, A. (1997). Sexual addiction. In *Substance abuse: A comprehensive textbook, 3rd ed.,* Lowinson, J., Ruiz, P., Millman, R. & Langrod, J., eds., 340–354. Baltimore: Williams & Wilkins.

Haack, M. R. & Adger H. (2002) Strategic plan for interdisciplinary faculty development. *Substance Abuse* 23 (3S), 345.

Hagemaster, J. N., Plumlee, A., Connors, H. & Sullivan, E. J. (1994). Integration of substance abuse content into undergraduate and graduate curricula. *Journal of Alcohol and Drug Education,* 40(1), 26–30.

Hall, M.J. & Popovich, J.R. (2000). *Summary: National hospital discharge summary advance data from vital and health statistics. no. 316.* Hyattsville, MD: National Center for Health Statistics.

Happell, B. & Taylor, C. (1999). Drug and alcohol education for nurses: have we examined the whole problem? *Journal of Addictions Nursing,* 11(4), 180–185.

Hoffman, A. L. & Heinemann, M. E. (1987). Substance abuse education in schools of nursing: A national survey. *Journal of Nursing Education,* 26(70), 282–287.

Huebner, H. (1993). *Endorphins, eating disorders, and other addictive behaviors.* New York: W. W. Norton.

Jacobs, D. F. (2000). Juvenile gambling in North America: An analysis of long term trends and future prospects. *Journal of Gambling Studies,* 16(2/3), 119–152.

Johnston, L. D., O'Malley, P. M., & Bachman, J. G. (2003). *Monitoring the future— National results on adolescent drug use: Overview of key findings, 2002.* NIH Publication No. 03-5374. Bethesda, MD: National Institute on Drug Abuse.

Korper, S. P., & Council, C. L. (Eds.). (2002). *Substance use by older adults: Estimates of future impact on the treatment systems* (DHHS Publication No. SMA 03-3763, Analytic Series A-21). Rockville, MD: Substance Abuse and Mental Health Services Administration, Office of Applied Studies.

Marcus, M.T. (1997). Faculty development and curricular change: A process and outcomes model for substance abuse education. *Journal of Professional Nursing,* 13:3, 168–177.

Marlatt, G. A. & Tapert. S.F. (1993). Harm reduction: Reducing the risks of addictive behaviors. In *Addictive behaviors across the life span: Prevention, treatment, and policy issues,* Baer, J.S., Marlatt, G.A. & McMahon, R.J., eds., 243–273. Newbury Park: CA: Sage.

Marlatt, G. A., & Witkiewitz, K. (2002). Harm reduction approaches to alcohol use: Health promotion, prevention, and treatment. *Addictive Behaviors, 27,* 867–886.

Martinez R. & Murphy-Parker, D.M. (2003). Examining the relationship of addiction education and beliefs of nursing students toward persons with alcohol problems. *Archives of Psychiatric Nursing,*17:4, 156–164.

McRee, B., Babor, T. & Church, O. (1991*). Project NEADA (Nursing education in alcohol and drug abuse).* University of Connecticut School of Nursing.

Mertens, I.L. & Van Gaal, L. (2000). Promising new approaches to the management of obesity. *Drugs,* 60 (1), 1–9.

Murphy-Parker, D. Kronenbitter, S. & Kronenbitter, R. (2003). National Student Nurses Association passes resolution in support of nursing school policies to assist and advocate nursing students experiencing impaired practice. *The Drug and Alcohol Professional,* 3 (2), 9–14.

Murray, C.J. & Lopez, A.D., eds. (1996*).* The global burden of disease. A comprehensive assessment of mortality and disability from diseases, injuries and risk factors in 1990 and projected to 2020. *Global Burden of Disease and Injury, Vol. 1.* Cambridge: Harvard University Press.

Naegle, M. & D'Areangelo, J. (1991). *Project SAEN (Substance Abuse Education in Nursing).* New York: New York University Division of Nursing.

National Gambling Impact and Policy Commission (NGIPC). (1999). *Final report—The national gambling impact study.* Washington, DC: NGIPC.

National Institute on Alcohol Abuse and Alcoholism. (1998). Drug abuse cost to society set at $97.7 billion, continuing steady increase since 1975. *NIDA Notes,* 13 (4), 1,12–13.

National Institute on Drug Abuse (NIDA) (2002a). *Diagnosis and treatment of drug abuse in family practice.* Public Health Service, National Institutes of Health (NIH), Department of Health and Human Services (DHHS), http://165.112.78.61/Diagnosis-Treatment/Diagnosis2.html, (accessed November 20, 2002).

National Institute on Drug Abuse (NIDA) (2002b). [Last updated September 13, 2002]. *Frequently asked questions*: What is drug addiction? Public Health Service, National Institutes of Health (NIH), Department of Health and Human Services (DHHS), http://www.drugabuse.gov/tools/FAQ.html, (accessed November 3, 2002).

National Nurses Society on Addiction (1993). Position paper: Addictive disorders among nurses and nursing students in academic settings. *Perspectives in Addictions Nursing,* 4(3), 1,7–8.

National Nurses Society on Addiction & American Nurses Association. (1989). *Standards of addiction nursing practice with selected diagnoses and criteria.* Kansas City, MO: American Nurses Association.

Nestler, E. J. (2001). Molecular neurobiology of addiction. *American Journal on Addictions,* 10, 201–217.

Pace, E. (2002). The employee assistance program as a model of care for an addicted colleague: Peer assistance, by nurses for nurses. *The Drug and Alcohol Professional,* 2 (3), 41–47.

Petrakis, I., & Krystal, J. (1997). Neuroscience: Implications for treatment. *Alcohol Health & Research World,* 21(2), 157–160.

Pirke, K. M. (1990). Central neurotransmitter disturbances in bulimia (nervosa). In *Bulimia nervosa: basic research, diagnosis and therapy,* Fichter, M. M., ed., 223–233. New York: John Wiley & Sons.

Rassool, G. H. (Ed.) (1998). *Substance use and misuse: Nature, context and clinical interventions.* Oxford: Blackwell Science.

Rassool, G. (2002). Substance misuse and mental health: An overview. *Nursing Standard,* 16 (50), 46–52.

Reisman, B.L. & Shrader, R.W. (1984). Effect of nurses' attitudes toward alcoholism on their referral rate for treatment. *Occupational Health Nursing* 32, 273–275.

Roberts, A. J., & Koob, G. F. (1997). The Neurobiology of addiction—An overview. *Alcohol Health & Research World*, 21(2), 101–108.

Ruden, R. A & Byalick, M. (1997) *The craving brain*. New York: HarperCollins.

Shaffer, H.J. & Hall, M.N. (2001). Updating and refining prevalence estimates of disordered gambling behavior in the United States and Canada. *Canadian Journal of Public Health,* 92(3), 168–172.

Sheehan, A. (1992). Nurses respond to substance abuse. *International Nurses Review,* 39(5), 141–144.

Smith, G.B. (1992). Attitudes of nurse managers and assistant nurse managers toward chemically impaired colleagues. *Image: Journal of Nursing Scholarship*, 24, 295–300.

Snow, D. (2000a) Managing patients with alcohol use disorders. *Lippincott's Primary Care Practice,* 4 (2), 131–148.

Snow, D (2000b) Neurobiology of addiction: The time has come. *Journal of Addictions Nursing,* 13 (3 &4), 3–4.

Starkey, P. J. (1980). Nurses' attitudes toward alcoholism. *AORN,* 31, 822.

Subcommittee on Health Services Research, National Advisory Council on Alcohol Abuse and Alcoholism. *Improving the delivery of alcohol treatment and prevention services: A national plan for alcohol health services research* (1997). Publication N. 97-4223. Bethesda, MD: National Institute on Alcohol Abuse and Alcoholism, National Institutes of Health, Department of Health and Human Services.

Substance Abuse and Mental Health Services Administration (SAMHSA). (2002). *Results from the 2001 National Household Survey on Drug Abuse: Volume I. Summary of national findings.* Office of Applied Studies, NHSDA Series H-17, DHHS Publication No. SMA 02-3758. Rockville, MD.

Sullivan, E. J. (1995). *Nursing care of clients with substance abuse.* St. Louis: Mosby.

Sullivan, E. J. & Handley, S. M. (1993). Nursing research on alcohol and drug abuse. In *Annual Review of Nursing Research. Vol.11,* Fitzpatrick, J.J., Taunton, R.L., & Benoliel, J.O., eds. New York: Springer.

Sullivan, E.F, & Fleming, M. (1997). A guide to substance abuse services for primary care clinicians. Treatment Improvement Protocol (TIP) Series 24.

Tamlyn, D.L. (1989). The effect of education on student nurses' attitudes toward alcoholics. *Canadian Journal of Nursing Research*, 21(3), 31–47.

Teutsch, S. (1992). A framework for assessing the effectiveness of disease and injury prevention. *Morbidity and Mortality Weekly Report*, 41 (RR-3), 1–12.

Trachtenberg, A. I., & Fleming, M. F. (1994). *Diagnosis and treatment of drug abuse in family practice*. Rockville, MD: National Institute of Drug Abuse.

Trinkoff, A.M., Eaton, W.W. & Anthony, J.C. (1991). The Prevalence of Substance Abuse Among Registered Nurses. *Nursing Research*, 40 (3), 172–75.

U.S. DHHS (Department of Health and Human Services). (2000). *Healthy People 2010*. National Center for Health Statistics. Hyattsville, MD: NCHS.

Velasquez, M. M.., Mauer, G. G., Crouch, C., & DiClemente, C. C. (2001). *Group treatment for substance abuse—A stages-of-change-therapy manual*. New York: Guilford Press.

Volberg, R.A. (1994). The prevalence and demographics of pathological gamblers: implications for public health: *American Journal of Public Health*, 84 (2), 237–41.

Vourakis, C. (1996). Addictions nursing practice is knowledge specific. *Journal of Addictions Nursing*, 8 (1), 2–3.

Wilcox, R.E. & Erickson, C.K. (2000). Neurological aspects of addictions. *Journal of Addictions Nursing*, 12 (3/4), 117–132.

Winick, C. (1997). Epidemiology. In *Substance abuse: A comprehensive textbook*. 3rd.ed., Lowinson, J., Ruiz, P., Millman, R. & Langrod, J., 10–16. Baltimore: Williams & Wilkins.

World Health Organization (1992). *The ICD-9. Classification of mental and behavioral disorders: Diagnostic criteria for research*. Geneva: World Health Organization.

World Health Organization (1993). *The ICD-10. Classification of mental and behavioral disorders: Diagnostic criteria for research*. Geneva: World Health Organization.

Appendix A
Specific Prevention Strategies

Information dissemination provides awareness and knowledge of the nature and extent of addictive behaviors, and their effects on persons, families, and communities. It also provides information to increase perception of risk, and information on healthy lifestyles.

Development of life coping skills seeks to affect critical life and social skills. Some of these include:

- decision-making,
- refusal,
- critical analysis,
- communication techniques,
- goal-setting,
- values clarification,
- problem-solving techniques,
- self-responsibility and self-care, and
- stress management and relaxation techniques.

Provision of alternatives involves targeted populations in activities that exclude addictive behaviors.

Community development aims to enhance the ability of the community to provide prevention and treatment services.

Advocacy for a healthy environment is used to set up or change written community standards, codes, and attitudes that influence and contribute to addiction.

Problem identification actually refers to secondary prevention, and involves screening and referral. After identification, this strategy calls for education and counseling of those who show evidence of being at risk for developing an addiction, and focusing on harm reduction strategies to prevent the development of additional problems related to addictions.

Primary prevention is utilized during the experimental/social stage of the process of addiction. Problem identification and other interventions are utilized during the problem use/abuse stage of the addictions process.

APPENDIX B
Motivational Interventions

According to CSAT:SAMHSA (1997) motivation is a key to change, multidimensional, a dynamic and fluctuating state, interactive, and influenced by the clinician's style.

In motivating a patient to change, the following strategies are recommended:

- Focus on the patient's strengths rather than their weaknesses.
- Respect the patient's autonomy and decisions.
- Provide individualized and patient-centered care.
- Do not depersonalize the patient by using labels like "addict".
- Develop a therapeutic partnership.
- Use empathy rather than authority or power.
- Focus on early intervention.
- Understand that intervention can happen in any setting.
- Recognize that addiction exists along a continuum.
- Recognize that many patients have more than one addiction.
- Recognize that many patients have other coexisting psychiatric or medical disorders that affect all stages of the change process.
- Accept goals that incorporate harm reduction, interim, incremental, and even temporary steps toward the ultimate goal of abstinence.
- Integrate interventions work with work done by other disciplines.

A motivational intervention is any clinical strategy designed to enhance patient motivation for change. It can include counseling, patient assessment, multiple sessions, or a 30-minute brief intervention.

The following elements of current motivational approaches have been found to be critical in prompting a person to change (SAMHSA, 1999b):

1) Use the FRAMES approach.

2) Incorporate decisional balance exercises.

3) Develop discrepancies for patients.

4) Use flexible pacing.

5) Establish personal contact with patients who are not actively in treatment.

The FRAMES approach consists of:

Feedback regarding personal risk or impairment following an assessment .

Responsibility for the change being placed with the patient.

Advice about changing—reducing or stopping the addictive behavior— given in a nonjudgmental manner.

Menu of self-directed change options and treatment alternatives offered to the patient.

Empathic counseling showing warmth, respect, and understanding.

Self-efficacy or optimistic empowerment engendered in the person to encourage change.

Research has shown that simple motivational interventions can be effective in encouraging patients to change, comply with treatment, or even return for more clinical appointments. Motivational interventions can take place in any setting, and offer great potential to reach persons with differing types of addictions from different cultural groups (CSAT:SAMHSA, 1997).

One of the key brief intervention activities is screening. Screening is usually done using brief written, oral, or computerized questionnaires. No screening instrument is effective with all persons. Therefore, it is important to consider a person's age, gender, race, ethnicity, and addiction before deciding on what screening instrument to use.

Screenings take approximately 10 to 15 minutes and are completed for the purposes of determining if a patient needs to be referred for a more in-depth assessment. Once the above considerations have been determined, it is important to use a screening instrument that has proven reliability and validity with the group of which the patient to be screened is a member. Many screening instruments exist that meet these criteria. They are easy to obtain in the literature, from books, or from addictions-related government clearinghouses.

APPENDIX C
Code of Ethics for Addictions Nurses

This code of ethics guides addictions nurses in maintaining a high level of competency in the provision of addictions nursing services.

As an addictions nurse, I acknowledge that my primary responsibility, regardless of any specific job title, is to meet my nursing responsibilities to the best of my ability. In implementing my responsibilities, I will adhere to the following principles:

I will remember that the care of the client is primary and I will ensure that he or she receives the highest possible level of quality care.

I will adhere to professional nursing standards and addictions nursing standards as currently defined.

I will understand and abide by the principles contained in the American Nurses Association Code for Nurses.

I will observe and maintain all rules of confidentiality.

I will conduct myself in such a professional manner as to promote the best interests of my clients and co-workers.

I will strive to increase my professional knowledge through continuing education.

I will seek and use professional supervision as a means of ensuring my competence to provide high quality care.

I will respect the boundaries of therapeutic relationships, and will not initiate or be the recipient of any personal or business relationships with clients.

I will strive to maintain my own personal health, so that I am fully capable of meeting my professional responsibilities, and will promptly seek assistance for any health problems or needs.

I will advocate on behalf of colleagues and nurses whose practice has become impaired as a result of addiction and/or psychological dysfunction, to ensure that they are treated fairly and appropriately.

I will respect the dignity and rights of all others, and will not discriminate against any client on the basis of race, gender, age, ethnicity, or religion.

I will act as an advocate for high quality addictions prevention and treatment within my workplace and my community.

I will recognize that the prevention of addictions is possible and I will engage in prevention activities within my worksite and my community.

~~~~

Published originally by National Nurses Society on Addictions (1995). Reprinted with permission of International Nurses Society on Addictions.

INDEX

A

Abuse stage of addiction, 8
  defined, 69
  See also Addiction, stages
Action (addiction behavior), 12
Addictions
  alcohol, 2, 3, 4, 5, 6
  associated diagnoses, 21
  as brain disorder, 6–7
  causes, 7
  characteristics, 5–10
  continuum of (well–illness), 7,
    16, 54, 79
  criteria for, 9–10
  defined, 5–6, 69
  diagnosis, 9–10
  drugs, 2, 3
  elderly and, 1, 4
  extent in United States, 2–4
  extent worldwide, 4
  food, 5, 6, 7, 29
  gambling, 5, 6, 7, 29
  genetics and, 6, 8, 28
  levels of use, 7
  mental illness and, 4, 12
  in nurses, 27, 29–30
  pain relievers, 3
  prevention, 10–11
  process, 7–9
  psychiatric disorders and, 7, 13,
    15, 18, 21, 23
  psychological effects, 18
  public misperceptions of, 6, 26
  public policy and, 11
  responses (actual or potential),
    16–20
  sex, 5, 6, 7, 29
  stages, 7–9
  tobacco, 2, 4
  tranquilizers, 3
  treatment, 12–14
  violence and, 4, 21
  See also Addictions nursing;
    Addictions nursing generalist
    level; Advanced Practice
    Registered Nurse in
    Addictions
Addictions nursing
  continuum of care, 10–14
  defined, 14–15
  historical background, 1–2
  phenomena of concern, 16–20
  practice environment, 15–16
  research, 1, 5–7, 8
  scope of practice, 14–30
  trends, 1–2
  See also Addiction; Addictions
    nursing generalist level;
    Advanced Practice Registered
    Nurse in Addictions
Addictions nursing advanced level.
  See Advanced Practice Registered
  Nurse in Addictions
Addictions Nursing Certification
  Board, 28
Addictions nursing generalist level
  assessment, 22, 31–32
  collaboration, 50
  collegiality, 48
  counseling, 42
  diagnosis, 33–34
  education, 21, 47
  ethics, 49
  evaluation, 43
  health promotion, health
    maintenance, and health
    teaching, 38
  implementation, 37–42

outcome identification, 35
pharmacological, biological, and
    complementary therapies, 40
planning, 36
performance appraisal, 46
qualifications, 21–22
quality of care, 45
research, 51
resource utilization, 52
scope of practice, 21–23
self-care and self-management, 39
skills, 22–23
therapeutic alliance, 37
therapeutic milieu, 41
See also Addiction; Addictions
    nursing; Advanced Practice
    Registered Nurse in
    Addictions
Addictive disorder, 7
    See also Addiction
Advanced Practice Registered Nurse
    (APRN) in Addictions,
        assessment, 53
    case management and
        coordination of care, 55
    consultation, 56
    diagnosis, 53
    education, 24, 63
    ethics, 65
    evaluation, 59
    health promotion, health
maintenance, and health teaching, 56
    implementation, 55
    interdisciplinary process, 66
    leadership, 64
    outcome identification, 54
    planning, 54
    prescriptive authority and
        treatment, 57
    psychotherapy and
        complementary therapy, 58

qualifications, 23
quality of care, 61
referral, 58
research, 67
scope of practice, 23–24
self-evaluation, 62
skills, 23–24
See also Addiction; Addictions
    nursing; Addictions nursing
    generalist level
Advocacy for patients and families, 25
    ethics and, 49
    prevention and, 81
Age-appropriate care. See Cultural
    competence
AlAnon, 14
Alcohol, 2, 3, 4, 5, 6, 27
Alcoholics Anonymous (AA), 14
American Nurses Association (ANA),
    1, 30
Amphetamines, 3
Analysis. See Critical thinking,
analysis, and synthesis
Anorexia. See Food disorders
Anxiety, 13, 14
Assessment
    brief intervention and, 12
    diagnosis and, 9, 33, 53
    education and, 26, 27
    motivational interventions and, 83
    objective data, 31
    outcome identification and, 54
    planning and, 54
    risk factors and, 10
    standard of care, 31–32, 53
    subjective data, 31
At risk use, 7, 26
    defined, 69
    See also Addiction, stages

B

Barbiturates, 3
Behaviors
    assessment and, 31
    conducive to addiction, 7
    counseling and, 42
    health promotion and, 25
    modification, 13
    motivation of change, 12, 81,
      83–84
    prevention and, 81
    psychotherapy and, 58
    recovery and, 14
    research, 29
    self-care and, 39
    stages of change, 12
    therapeutic alliance and, 37
    therapy, 13
Best practices, 11
    assessment and, 53
    consultation and, 56
    implementation and, 55
    outcome identification and, 54
    pharmacological, biological, and
      complementary therapies and,
      40
    planning and, 36
    psychotherapy and, 58
    therapeutic milieu and, 41
Biological vulnerability to addiction,
    7, 10
Brain. *See* Neurology
Brief intervention, 11–12, 80
    education and, 26
    See also Continuum of
      addictions nursing care
Bulimia. *See* Food disorders

C

Cancer, 21
Care of Clients with Addictions:
    Dimensions of Nursing Practice, 1
Care recipient. *See* Patient
Care standards. *See* Standards of care
Case management and coordination
    of care
    for addicted nurses, 30
    advanced practice and, 24, 25
    planning and, 36
    standard of care, 55
    treatment and, 13
Center for Substance Abuse
    Prevention (CSAP), 11, 26
    See also Substance Abuse and
      Mental Health Services
      Administration
Center for Substance Abuse
    Treatment, 7
    See also Substance Abuse and
      Mental Health Services
      Administration
Certification and credentialing,
    27–28, 29–30
    education and, 47
    prescriptive authority and, 57
    psychotherapy and, 58
    quality of care and, 61
Certified Addictions Registered
    Nurse (CARN), 27–28
    See also Addictions nursing
      general practice
Certified Addictions Registered
    Nurse-Advanced Practice (CARN-
    AP), 28
    See also Advanced Practice
      Registered Nurse in Addictions
Characteristics of addiction, 5–10
Children. *See* Family
Client. *See* Patient
Clinical settings. *See* Practice settings

Cocaine, 3

Cocaine Anonymous (CA), 14

Code of Ethics for Addictions Nurses, 25, 85–86
   See also Ethics

Code of Ethics for Nurses with Interpretive Statements, 49
   See also Ethics

Cognitive effects of addiction, 18–19
   diagnosis and, 33
   health teaching and, 38
   See also Phenomena of concern to addictions nursing

Collaboration
   counseling and, 42
   interdisciplinary process and, 66
   planning and, 36
   research and, 51
   standard of professional performance, 50
   therapeutic milieu and, 41
   See also Interdisciplinary healthcare teams

Collegiality
   leadership and, 64
   performance appraisal and, 46
   self-evaluation and, 62
   standard of professional performance, 48

Communication
   assessment and, 31
   collegiality and, 48
   prevention and, 81
   research and, 29, 49, 67
   self-evaluation and, 62

Community health, 15, 19–20
   advance practice and, 24
   advocacy for, 25
   assessment and, 31
   collaboration and, 49
   diagnosis and, 34
   health teaching and, 38

   research and, 51
   self-care and, 39
   strategies, 81
   therapeutic milieu and, 41

Competence assessment. *See* Certification and credentialing

Complementary therapies, 13, 58
   See also Holistic care; Pharmacological, biological, and complementary therapies

Compulsions and addictions, 6, 25, 31

Confidentiality
   counseling and, 42
   ethics and, 49
   See also Ethics

Consolidated Association of Nurses in Substance Abuse International, 28

Consultation
   interdisciplinary process and, 66
   research and, 67
   standard of care, 56

Contemplation (addiction behavior), 12

Continuity of care
   collaboration and, 50
   outcome identification and, 35

Continuum of addiction (well–illness), 7, 16, 54, 79

Continuum of addictions nursing care, 10–14, 15
   brief (early) intervention, 11–12, 80
   prevention, 10–11
   recovery, 14
   treatment, 12–14

Co-occurring disorder (defined), 69
   See also Mental illness/ substance abuse (MISA)

Coordination of care. *See* Case management and coordination of care; Interdisciplinary healthcare teams

Coping skills, 14
　　assessment and, 31
　　counseling and, 42
　　health teaching and, 38
　　prevention and, 81
　　self-care and, 39
　　therapeutic alliance and, 37
Cost control,
　　ethics and, 65
　　outcome identification and, 35, 54
　　pharmacological, biological, and
　　　complementary therapies and,
　　　40
　　in prevention of addiction, 11
　　quality of care and, 61
　　referral and, 58
　　resource utilization and, 52
Cost-effectiveness. *See* Cost control
Counseling, 12, 13
　　for addicted nurses, 30
　　motivational interventions and, 83
　　skills at general practice level, 22
　　standard of care, 42
Crack, 3
Craving, 14
　　defined, 69
Credentialing. *See* Certification and
　　credentialing
Criteria,
　　assessment, 31–32, 53
　　case management and
coordination of care, 55
　　collaboration, 50
　　collegiality, 48
　　consultation, 56
　　counseling, 42
　　diagnosis, 33–34, 53
　　education, 47, 63
　　ethics, 49, 65
　　evaluation, 43, 59

　　health promotion, health
　　　maintenance, and health
　　　teaching, 38, 56
　　implementation, 37–42, 55
　　interdisciplinary process, 66
　　leadership, 64
　　outcome identification, 35, 54
　　pharmacological, biological, and
　　　complementary therapies, 40
　　planning, 36, 54
　　performance appraisal, 46
　　prescriptive authority and
　　　treatment, 57
　　psychotherapy and
　　　complementary therapy, 58
　　quality of care, 45, 61
　　referral, 58
　　research, 51, 67
　　resource utilization, 52
　　self-care and self-management, 39
　　self-evaluation, 62
　　therapeutic alliance, 37
　　therapeutic milieu, 41
Criteria of addiction, 9–10
Critical thinking, analysis, and
　synthesis
　　assessment and, 32
　　case management and, 55
　　diagnosis and, 53
　　health promotion and, 56
　　prescriptive authority and, 57
　　quality of care and, 45, 61
Cultural competence
　　advance practice and, 24
　　assessment and, 31
　　education and, 27
　　ethics and, 49
　　health teaching and, 38, 56

outcome identification and, 35, 54
planning and, 36
self-care and, 39
therapeutic milieu and, 41
Culture and addiction, 6, 10

D
Data collection,
  assessment and, 31, 53
  quality of care and, 45
  research and, 51
Decision-making
  consultation and, 56
  diagnosis and, 33
  planning and, 54
  prescriptive authority and, 57
Dependency stage of addiction, 6, 7
  defined, 69
  treatment and, 13
  See also Addiction, stages
Depression, 4, 14
Detoxification, 12, 13
  defined, 69
  diagnosis and, 34
Developmental levels, 14
  assessment and, 31
  diagnosis and, 33
  health teaching and, 38, 56
  planning and, 36
  self-care and, 39
Diagnosis
  of addiction, 9–10
  alcohol-related, 5
  assessment and, 53
  criteria, 9–10
  differential, 27, 53
  education and, 27
  evaluation and, 43, 59
  outcome identification and, 35, 54
  planning and, 54
  prescriptive authority and, 57

quality of care and, 61
standard of care, 33–34, 53
*Diagnostic and Statistical Manual of
  Mental Disorders, 4th Edition Text
  Revision* (DMS-IV-TR), 9, 33, 53
Disease Adjusted Life Years (DALYs), 4
Documentation
  assessment and, 32
  counseling and, 42
  diagnosis and, 34
  education and, 47
  evaluation and, 43
  health teaching and, 38
  implementation and, 37
  outcome identification and, 35
  pharmacological, biological, and
    complementary therapies and,
    40
  planning and, 36, 54
  self-care and, 39
  therapeutic alliance and, 37
  therapeutic milieu and, 41
Drug abuse, 2, 3
Drug and Alcohol Nurses Association, 1
Dual diagnosis. *See* Mental
  illness/substance abuse (MISA)

E
Early intervention. *See* Brief
  intervention
Eating disorders, 5, 6, 7, 8
  defined, 69
Economic issues. *See* Cost control
Ecstasy (MDMA), 3
Education of addictions nurses
  collegiality and, 48
  curriculum, 26–27
  importance of, 26
  interdisciplinary process and, 66
  prevention and, 11
  prescriptive authority and, 57

research and, 29, 67
standard of professional
    performance, 47, 63
See also Professional
    development
Education of patients and families
    ethics and, 65
    health promotion and, 56
    planning and, 36
    prescriptive authority and, 57
    psychotherapy and, 58
    resource utilization and, 52
    therapeutic milieu and, 41
    See also Family; Health
        promotion, health
        maintenance, and health
        teaching; Patient
Elderly and addictions, 1, 4, 15
Emotional aspects of addiction, 5, 8,
    10, 33, 34
    assessment data, 31
    children's emotional
        development, 19
    See also Family; Psychological
        aspects of addiction
Environmental vulnerability to
    addiction, 7, 10
Ethics
    codes, 25, 49, 85–86
    counseling and, 42
    implementation and, 37
    peer assistance and, 29
    standard of professional
        performance, 49, 65
    therapeutic alliance and, 37
Evaluation
    counseling and, 42
    pharmacological, biological, and
        complementary therapies and,
        40
    prescriptive authority and, 57
    psychotherapy and, 58

research and, 67
self-care and, 39
standard of care, 43, 59
Evidence-based practice, 15, 26, 29
    assessment and, 53
    diagnosis and, 33
    education and, 47
    evaluation and, 59
    implementation and, 37, 55
    outcome identification and, 35, 54
    planning and, 36, 54
    prescriptive authority and, 57
    psychotherapy and, 58
    quality of care and, 61
    therapeutic milieu and, 41
    See also Research
Experimentation stage of addiction, 8
    See also Addiction, stages
Extent of addictions, 2–5

F
Family
    addiction and, 6, 19
    addictions nursing and, 15
    assessment and, 31
    collaboration and, 50
    counseling and, 42
    diagnosis and, 33
    evaluation and, 43
    health teaching and, 38
    outcome identification and, 35
    pharmacological, biological, and
        complementary therapies and,
        40
    psychotherapy and, 58
    resource utilization and, 52
    support programs, 14
    See also Phenomena of concern
        to addictions nursing
Financial issues, 1, 14
    See also Cost control

Food disorders, 5, 6, 7, 8, 29
FRAMES (Feedback, Responsibility, Advice, Menu, Empathy, Self-efficacy) approach to motivation, 84

G

GamAnon, 14
Gamblers Anonymous (GA), 14
Gambling, 4, 6, 7, 8, 29
Genetic predisposition to addiction, 6, 8, 28
Global Burden of Disease (GBD), 4

H

Hallucinogens, 3
Harm/risk reduction (defined), 69
Health promotion, health maintenance, and health teaching, 15–16, 24–25
    diagnosis and, 33
    pharmacological, biological, and complementary therapies and, 40
    planning and, 36, 54
    psychotherapy and, 58
    standard of care, 38, 56
    therapeutic alliance and, 37
Healthcare policy
    addictions nursing and, 1
    leadership and, 64
    quality of care and, 45
    research and, 51
Healthcare providers
    addictions nursing and, 15
    advance practice and, 24
    assessment and, 32
    case management and, 55
    collaboration and, 50
    collegiality and, 48
    diagnosis and, 33
    evaluation and, 43

interdisciplinary process and, 66
    pharmacological, biological, and complementary therapies and, 40
    planning and, 54
    quality of care and, 61
    referral and, 58
    therapeutic milieu and, 41
    See also Interdisciplinary healthcare teams
Hepatitus, 13, 17, 21
Heroin, 3
HIV/AIDS, 4, 13, 17, 21
Holistic care, 9, 13, 15
Human resources. See Professional development

I

Implementation
    patient and, 23
    planning and, 23
    quality of care and, 45
    research and, 51
    standard of care, 37, 55
Impulse-control disorder (defined), 70
Information. See Data collection
Inhalants, 3
Interdisciplinary healthcare
    assessment and, 32
    collegiality and, 48
    counseling and, 42
    education and, 47
    evaluation and, 43
    implementation and, 37
    outcome identification and, 35, 54
    planning and, 36, 54
    quality of care and, 45
    recovery and, 14
    standard of professional performance, 66
    See also Collaboration

International Classification of
Diseases, 33, 53
International Nurses Society on
Addictions, 28, 30
Interventions
    assessment and, 53
    brief (early), 11–12, 26, 80
    counseling and, 42
    education and, 27
    ethics and, 49
    evaluation and, 43, 59
    health promotion and, 56
    implementation and, 37, 55
    motivational, 81, 83–84
    pharmacological, biological, and
      complementary therapies and,
      40
    planning and, 36, 54
    prescriptive authority and, 57
    prevention and, 10–11
    recovery and, 14, 16
    research and, 51
    self-care and, 39
    therapeutic alliance and, 37
    in treatment, 13

J
Journal of Addictions Nursing, 29, 67

L
Laws, statutes, and regulations
    counseling and, 42
    ethics and, 49
    performance appraisal and, 46
    prescriptive authority and, 57
    self-evaluation and, 62
    therapeutic milieu and, 41
    See also Ethics
Leadership
    advance practice and, 24

quality of care and, 61
standard of professional
    performance, 64
Legal effects of addiction, 20
    See also Phenomena of concern
      to addictions nursing
Legal issues. *See* Laws, statutes, and
    regulations
Licensing. *See* Certification and
    credentialing
Low risk use, 7
    defined, 70
    See also Addiction, stages

M
Maintenance (addiction behavior), 12
Marijuana, 3
Measurement criteria. *See* Criteria
Medication, 12, 13
    diagnosis and, 34
    education and, 26
Mental illness and addiction
    diagnosis and, 33–34
    incidence of, 4
    pharmacological, biological, and
      complementary therapies and,
      40
    treatment, 12, 13
Mental illness/substance abuse
    (MISA), 13, 15, 21
Mentoring
    advance practice and, 24
    collegiality and, 48
    leadership and, 64
Methamphetamines, 3
Misuse stage of addiction, 8
    See also Addiction, stages
Monitoring the Future, 2, 3
Motivation of behavioral change,
    12, 14
    therapeutic alliance and, 37

Motivational intervention, 83–84
Multidisciplinary healthcare. *See* Interdisciplinary healthcare

N
NarAnon, 14
Narcotics Anonymous (NA), 14
National Hospital Discharge Survey, 5
National Household Survey on Drug Abuse, 2–4
National Institute on Alcohol Abuse and Alcoholism, 5, 26, 28–29
National Institute on Drug Abuse, 5, 6, 26, 28–29
National Institutes of Health, 28–29, 67
National Nurses Society on Addictions, 1
National Student Nurses Association, 30
Neurobiology
    addiction and, 6–7
    education and, 26
    planning and, 36
    research, 28
Nicotine, 6
North American Nursing Diagnosis Association (NANDA) Nursing Diagnosis Classification, 33
Nurses with addictions, 27, 29–30
Nursing care standards. *See* Standards of care
Nursing standards. *See* Standards of care; Standards of professional performance

O
Objective data, 31
Office for Substance Abuse Prevention, 26
    See also Center for Substance Abuse Prevention (CSAP)

Outcome identification
    standard of care, 35, 54
    See also Outcomes
Outcomes
    collaboration and, 50
    diagnosis and, 34
    ethics and, 49, 65
    evaluation and, 43, 59
    implementation and, 37
    performance appraisal and, 46
    planning and, 36, 54
    psychotherapy and, 58
    quality of care and, 45
    self-evaluation and, 62
    See also Outcome identification
Overeaters Anonymous, 14
Oxycontin, 3

P
Pain management, 21
Pain relievers, 3
Parents. *See* Family
Patient
    assessment and, 31, 32
    case management and, 55
    collaboration and, 50
    consultation and, 56
    counseling and, 42
    diagnosis and, 33
    ethics and, 49, 65
    evaluation and, 43
    health teaching and, 38
    implementation and, 23, 37
    motivational interventions, 83
    outcome identification and, 35, 54
    performance appraisal and, 46
    pharmacological, biological, and complementary therapies and, 40
    planning and, 23, 36, 54
    psychotherapy and, 58
    quality of care and, 45, 61

relationship with addictions
  nurse, 22, 65
rights, 25
responsibilities, 7, 39, 56
resource utilization and, 52
respect for,
self-care and, 39
therapeutic milieu and, 41
See also Family
PCP (phencyclidine), 3
Peer assistance. *See* Nurses with
  addictions
Peer review
  collegiality and, 48
  performance appraisal and, 46
  self-evaluation and, 62
Performance appraisal
  collegiality and, 48
  self-evaluation and, 62
  standard of professional
    performance, 46
Pharmacologic agents. *See*
  Prescriptive authority
Pharmacological, biological, and
  complementary therapies
  standard of care, 40
  See also Medication
Phenomena of concern to addictions
  nursing, 16–20
  cognitive effects, 18–19
  effects on family, 19
  legal effects, 20
  physiological effects, 17
  psychological effects, 18
  spiritual effects, 18
  workplace effects, 20
Physiological dependence (defined),
  70
Physiological effects of addiction, 17
  See also Phenomena of concern
    to addictions nursing

Planning
  counseling and, 42, 56
  consultation and, 56
  diagnosis and, 34
  evaluation and, 43, 59
  implementation and, 37
  outcome identification and, 35
  patient and, 23
  performance appraisal and, 46
  quality of care and, 45
  research and, 51
  standard of care, 36, 54
  treatment and, 12, 23
Policy. *See* Healthcare policy
Practice settings, 5, 9
  general practice, 22
  treatment and, 13
Preceptors. *See* Mentoring
Pre-contemplation (addiction
  behavior), 12
Preparation (addiction behavior), 12
Prescriptive authority and treatment
  implementation and, 55
  standard of care, 57
Prevention of addiction, 10–11
  counseling and, 42
  defined, 10, 70
  diagnosis and, 33
  education and, 11, 24, 26, 27
  health promotion and, 56
  prescriptive authority and, 57
  primary, 81
  secondary, 81
  strategies, 81
  See also Continuum of
    addictions nursing care
Principles of Drug Addiction
  Treatment, 12–13
Privacy. *See* Confidentiality
Problem use stage of addiction, 7
  See also Addiction, stages

Professional development,
    collegiality and, 48
    education and, 63
    leadership and, 64
    research and, 51, 67
    self-evaluation and, 62
    See also Education; Leadership
Professional performance. See
    Standards of professional
    performance
Protective factors, 10
Psychiatric disorders
    incidence of, 4
    co-occurrence with addictions,
        7, 13, 15, 18, 21, 23
    in nurses, 29, 30
Psychological aspects of addiction,
    10, 18, 15, 21, 33, 34, 41
    See also Emotional aspects of
        addiction
Psychological effects of addiction, 18
    See also Phenomena of concern
        to addictions nursing
Psychotherapy and complementary
    therapy
    standard of care, 58
Public policy on addiction, 11

Q

Quality of care
    advance practice and, 24
    consultation and, 56
    leadership and, 64
    standard of professional
        performance, 45, 61

R

Recipient of care. See Patient
Recovery stage of addiction
    addictions nurse and, 22

health teaching and, 38
treatment and, 13, 14, 23
See also Addiction, stages;
    Continuum of addictions
    nursing care
Referral, 9, 27
    ethics and, 49
    counseling and, 42
    standard of care, 58
Regulatory issues. See Laws, statutes,
    and regulations
Relapse stage of addiction, 6
    addiction behavior, 12
    defined, 70
    health teaching and, 38
    during treatment, 13
    prevention, 14
    See also Addiction, stages
Remission (defined), 70
Research
    in addictions nursing, 1, 5–7, 8,
        24, 25, 28–29
    assessment and, 32, 53
    consultation and, 56
    education and, 47, 63
    evaluation and, 59
    health promotion and, 56
    implementation and, 55
    importance of, 26
    interdisciplinary process and, 66
    outcome identification and, 35, 54
    performance appraisal and, 46
    pharmacological, biological, and
        complementary therapies and,
        40
    planning and, 54
    prescriptive authority and, 57
    psychotherapy and, 58
    quality of care and, 61

standard of professional
   performance, 51
  See also Evidence-based practice
Resource utilization, 25
  ethics and, 49
  outcome identification and, 35
  standard of professional
performance, 52
Risk. *See* Low risk; At risk
Risk factors, 10
  diagnosis and, 33
  health teaching and, 38
Rohypnol, 4

S
Safety assurance, 9, 25, 40, 41
  ethics, interventions, and 37
  implementation and, 37
  quality of care and, 45, 61
  resource utilization and, 52
Scientific findings. *See* Evidence-
  based practice; Research
Scope of practice, 14–30
  advanced level, 23–24
  generalist level, 21–23
Screening, 84
Self-care and self-management,
  diagnosis and, 33
  recovery and, 14
  standard of care, 39
Self-evaluation
  standard of professional
   performance, 62
Self-help groups, 14
  counseling and, 42
  self-care and, 39
Settings. *See* Practice settings
Sex Anonymous (SA), 14
Sexual addiction, 5, 6, 7, 29
Sexually-transmitted diseases, 21
Significant others. *See* Family

Social effects of addiction, 10, 19–20
Social use. *See* Experimentation
stage of addiction
Spiritual health, 14, 18
  assessment and, 31
  diagnosis and, 33, 34
  health teaching and, 38
  outcome identification and, 35
  therapeutic milieu and, 41
  See also Cultural Competence;
   Phenomena of concern to
   addictions nursing
Stages of addiction, 7–9
  dependence, 8
  experimentation, 7, 8
  problem use, 8
  recovery, 8–9
  relapse, 9
Standards of care
  assessment, 31–32, 53
  case management and
   coordination of care, 55
  consultation, 56
  counseling, 42
  diagnosis, 33–34, 53
  evaluation, 43, 59
  health promotion, health
   maintenance, and health
   teaching, 38, 56
  implementation, 37–42, 55
  outcome identification, 35, 54
  pharmacological, biological, and
   complementary therapies, 40
  planning, 36, 54
  prescriptive authority and
   treatment, 57
  psychotherapy and
   complementary therapy, 58
  referral, 58
  self-care and self-management, 39
  therapeutic alliance, 37
  therapeutic milieu, 41

Standards of Addictions Nursing Practice with Selected Diagnoses and Criteria (1987), 1
Standards of practice. *See* Standards of care
Standards of professional performance
  collaboration, 50
  collegiality, 48
  education, 47, 63
  ethics, 49, 65
  interdisciplinary process, 66
  leadership, 64
  performance appraisal, 46
  quality of care, 45, 61
  research, 51, 67
  resource utilization, 52
  self-evaluation, 62
Strategies for prevention of addiction, 81
Stress management, 13
Subjective data, 31
Substance abuse (defined), 70
Substance Abuse and Mental Health Services Administration (SAMHSA), 7, 11
Substance dependence (defined), 70
Substance misuse (defined), 71
Substance use disorder (SUD) (defined), 71
Substances (defined), 71
Support programs, 14
  counseling and, 42
  self-care and, 39
Synthesis. *See* Critical thinking, analysis, and synthesis

T
Teaching. *See* Education; Health promotion, health maintenance, and health teaching

Teams and teamwork. *See* Interdisciplinary healthcare
Therapeutic alliance, 22
  standard of care, 37
Therapeutic milieu, 22
  standard of care, 41
Therapy, 13
  See also Interventions
Tobacco, 2, 4
Tolerance, 6, 9
  defined, 71
Traffic accidents, 4
Tranquilizers, 3
Treatment, 12–14
  See also Continuum of addictions nursing care
Tuberculosis, 13, 21

V
Violence and addiction, 4, 21
Vulnerability to addiction, 7, 10

W
Well–illness addictions continuum, 7, 16, 54, 79
Withdrawal, 6, 9
  education and, 26
  defined, 71
  pharmacological, biological, and complementary therapies and, 40
  treatment and, 13
Workplace
  assessment and, 31
  effects of addiction, 20
  See also Phenomena of concern to addictions nursing
World Health Organization (WHO), 4